How
Would You Like
Your Eggs?

A Journal about Life with Unexplained Infertility

Debora Krizak

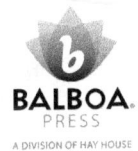

BALBOA
PRESS

A DIVISION OF HAY HOUSE

Balboa Press books may be ordered through booksellers or by contacting:

Balboa Press
A Division of Hay House
1663 Liberty Drive
Bloomington, IN 47403
www.balboapress.com.au
1-(877) 407-4847

ISBN: 978-1-4525-1020-0 (sc)
ISBN: 978-1-4525-1021-7 (e)

Because of the dynamic nature of the Internet, any web addresses or
links contained in this book may have changed since publication and
may no longer be valid. The views expressed in this work are solely those
of the author and do not necessarily reflect the views of the publisher,
and the publisher hereby disclaims any responsibility for them.

The author of this book does not dispense medical advice or prescribe the use
of any technique as a form of treatment for physical, emotional, or medical
problems without the advice of a physician, either directly or indirectly. The
intent of the author is only to offer information of a general nature to help
you in your quest for emotional and spiritual well-being. In the event you use
any of the information in this book for yourself, which is your constitutional
right, the author and the publisher assume no responsibility for your actions.

Any people depicted in stock imagery provided by Thinkstock are models,
and such images are being used for illustrative purposes only.
Certain stock imagery © Thinkstock.

Printed in the United States of America

Balboa Press rev. date: 05/28/2013

Disclaimer

This publication is designed to provide support, educational and general information. It is not meant to substitute, in any way, for medical advice. The author has put forward her best effort to provide information on the topic, but there is no warranty with respect to the accuracy or completeness of this publication. As developments in this area continue, some of the references may be out date by the time you read this publication.

The situation and advice provided to the author in this publication may not be applicable or advisable for your particular circumstance. Consult with a medical professional when and where appropriate. The author is not responsible or liable for any damages, including, but not limited to special, consequential, incidental, or other damages arising directly or indirectly from this publication.

In some cases identifying details of people associated with the author have been changed, in others appropriate permission has been sought from the individuals involved.

Any trade names of medications are used for informational purposes only.

FOR THE 'NUGGETS'

FOREWORD

"So, when are you guys going to have kids?" It is a question usually asked with nothing more sinister than friendly curiosity. But I'll let you into a secret—for some of us it's a question that can cut like a knife and can trigger feelings of self-blame, guilt, shame, loss of control and anger.

It's one of many. We've all heard them. Some of us have even asked them: *"Don't you want kids?" "What's wrong with you?"* . . . the list goes on. They seem never-ending and there is no easy answer.

There might be many reasons why we have waited to start a family—to set ourselves up financially, moving cities, buying a house or only just finding 'Mr Right' (or ourselves for that matter). But when you are desperately longing for a baby, wondering whether you will ever hold one in your arms, the questions sting.

It's not like you don't have a whole list of questions of your own; *"My friends all seem to be able to get pregnant immediately, so why isn't it happening for us?"* *"Is it my fault?"* *"How many more disappointments can we take?"* *"Will we have to give up on our dream?"* It can become all consuming and impact on every aspect of your life and relationships.

Some people prefer to keep their experiences to themselves, feeling safer trying to lock themselves away from the fertile world.

Me? I was more likely to enlighten those who asked insensitive questions—and give details. We're talking charting cervical mucus, sex on cue, wooden fertility dolls, swallowing foul tasting Chinese herbs. It was definitely enough to make most people think twice about asking me anything ever again.

Even though one in six Australian couples experience some kind of fertility problem, it can be an incredibly isolating condition. I, like many other women, found solace in connecting through online forums—where you can pour out your heart to virtual strangers who cannot see your tears, but can feel your pain.

Looking back on my journey, there were a few pivotal moments although I didn't recognise them at the time because my vision was often clouded by grief and blinded by my deep longing to have a baby. The red polka dotted dress; the kind stranger, a flight to Singapore and the persistent owners of the little B & B we escaped to in the midst of our IVF treatment. All of them piece together a long line of dots throughout my years of struggling to conceive.

I was immersed in my secret life—my perpetual state of PUPO (pregnant until proven otherwise)—repeatedly promising myself that the furtively purchased pregnancy tests would only be used if completely justified, then sneaking off to pee on a stick . . . and then another one just in case.

Robbed of the enjoyment of planning for a baby, everything became covert—a conspiracy shared with my husband and my mother.

Then came the emotional rollercoaster of IVF, while putting on a brave face for a continuous line of baby showers for other people.

My journey took me from almost losing all hope, to the joy of finally becoming a mum. It was such an unexpected, unpredictable story. And it is one I now feel compelled to share—to try to shine a light on a common but misunderstood condition and to be an advocate for other women still isolated in their own infertility bubbles. To start a conversation in a world that appears to prefer to ignore the issue of infertility.

I promise to expose the full myriad of emotions and share heartbreaking experiences, as well as offer hope when it appears that all the statistics were lined up against us.

Everyone's experience of infertility is different and we all have our own unique journey. Different doctors have different approaches. But I feel, as patients, infertility is uniting and my sole purpose for writing this book is to provide support and guidance no matter what the outcome is.

My experience saw me embark on treatment at two different fertility clinics, with very different approaches. As time passed, I realised there was no greater power than education. I informed myself about the subtle differences in treatments and armed myself with as much knowledge and research as possible.

Sometimes, it takes more than two people to make a pregnancy and it can take time. It doesn't always mean the diagnosis is infertility. Make an appointment to see a doctor and discuss any concerns you may have. Being well informed is the key to knowing what options are available to you.

I'm approaching this book like a journal so I can keep it open and honest. I'll share with you the good, the bad and the funny side of some of the hurdles I encountered. Heck knows we all need a good laugh from time to time. It's often been the only thing to get me through.

I realise infertility is not a laughing matter, so I have worked with Genea, World Leaders in Fertility to include some of the more technical details—which I hope you will find very helpful.

If this book can help lighten the load of the grieving process you experience on your own personal journey, or be a reference for someone close to you, then together we can help others understand. Best of luck and enjoy.

Debora

Debora Krizak

CHAPTER 1

Where did the time go?

"Each human being has exactly the same number of hours and minutes every day. Rich people can't buy more hours. Scientists can't invent new minutes. And you can't save time to spend it on another day. Even so, time is amazingly fair and forgiving. No matter how much time you've wasted in the past, you still have an entire tomorrow."
—DENIS WAITELY

Year 1, August—
Time flies when you're having fun

I was emptying out my bedside drawers the other day when I stumbled across a half empty box of oral contraceptives. It seems like a lifetime ago since I took them. I flipped the packet around to have a look at the issue date—five years ago. That's how long I had been off the pill. I'd never really thought of it before that moment.

My husband Fez and I have enjoyed a normal sex life and, like most couples, have taken a few risks from time to time which eventually resorted to us doing away with contraception altogether. We have been in the mindset that we would let nature take its course and not think about things too much. 'Let it be a surprise if we get pregnant,' we said, relishing all the romantic notions that go along with the idea. Five years later and nothing. Where has the time gone?

I've always been ambitious and career-oriented, and so opted for a Performing Arts Degree straight out of high school before beginning to dabble in the entertainment industry. I had my heart set on becoming a dancer. Unfortunately no-one was honest enough to gently guide me away from that profession when physicality and natural talent were clearly not on my side.

So I blindly went ahead and studied dance as a major at Adelaide University, continuing to be unfulfilled. That is, until I answered an ad in the Uni paper. The ad was for a young singer to front a local covers band to work with a professional group of musicians. I went along to the audition and got the job. It wasn't long before I was gigging around town and making a small name for myself. I was never trained professionally, but singing was always something that came easily to me. I guess I took it for granted a little. I had a natural love of it and so began to revel in my new found talent. In no time, dance became a distant interest as I was able to make myself a nice income singing while all of my fellow Uni students slogged it out waiting tables on weekends. After graduating I decided to make singing my profession and hung up my dancing shoes once and for all.

Living in Adelaide was a great place to hone my skills as a performer. Whilst making a name for myself (a big fish in a small pond), I spent the first few years of my twenties desperately trying to carve my own little niche and strive for goals that had previously been just a figment of my imagination. At 23, I was hosting *The Music Shop*, a national TV children's show and was fortunate enough to buy my first property—a two bedroom unit in Hectorville, about 8 minutes from the city. I'd set myself up and was itching to venture further into the bright lights of the entertainment industry. I had my sights set on musical theatre but for that I needed to be based in either Melbourne or Sydney—so I began to psyche myself up for a move.

My moving plans came unravelled pretty quickly when I answered another newspaper ad to audition for a well-known covers band in Adelaide called 'Chunky Custard'. I got the job and dedicated the next seven years of my life to touring exclusively with this act and living it up as a 'rock and roll artist'. It was everything I could have dreamed of: good money, travel, great exposure and, above all else, I met the man I would marry.

Fez was a co-director of the business, which went on to become one of the biggest cover bands to come out of Australia. Five years after our first meeting, on a cold, rainy day in March, we took our vows in a quaint little church at Eagle on the Hill in the Adelaide Hills. Then, a year later, with success in our wake, we decided to leave our comfortable home town and spread our wings. My 'move' was finally a reality, Fez and I were to start an entertainment business of our own in the bright lights of the harbour city—Sydney.

We arrived in Sydney brimming with expectations of what was around the corner for us. I was a 29-year-old aspiring singer/actress and my husband Fez was a musician/entertainment agent. We made a great team and were going to thrive bringing new projects to fruition together. We had saved enough money prior to leaving Adelaide to afford six months' worth of Sydney rent. We knew the savings wouldn't get us much further than that, but it helped us to establish ourselves in a tough musical market and to gain a reputation from prominent Sydney entertainment agents. To get the ball rolling we auditioned a number of Sydney musos and, before long, had our own four-piece covers band working the nightly slog of nightclubs and bars. The pay was minimal, but we were there. The band was called 'Tall Pop Syndrome'. Fez played keyboards and I was up front on vocals. It quickly became one of the top five corporate covers acts in Sydney and franchised into three different line ups of the same band to be able to cope with the demand. Nothing was impossible. Not for us.

In moving states and starting afresh, Fez and I had taken a leap of faith in our relationships and our careers. Leaving Adelaide had its drawbacks, most of them emotional. I'd left behind my small, close-knit family of two older brothers and a mum and dad who were still very much in love after 40 years of marriage. Fez also left his family behind—his mum and dad, with whom he had only just reconnected after a messy divorce, and his brother, eight years his junior, who often looked to Fez as a fatherly figure. Family was important to us, and there was nowhere to fall if things didn't work out for us in Sydney.

But as hard as moving to Sydney was for us, we felt that if we didn't do it when we did, then we'd live and die in suburban Adelaide—something neither of us wanted. We wanted our families to be proud of what we were doing, embrace our new found courage, and see that we could do it alone. At the airport on the day we left Adelaide, I recall the awkward silence as we waited to board our plane for the new life that awaited us in Sydney. My mum managed to keep a brave face but it wasn't until much later that I realised the impact it must have had on her, when her only daughter moved so many kilometres away.

Flying over the Adelaide plains that day, we said 'goodbye' to life as we had known it and 'hello' to a whole new world of possibility. I had dreams of treading the boards with the best in the industry, performing on the big stage with the bright lights of the theatre and an ensemble of like-minded, creative people around me. I longed for recognition for all the years I'd slogged it out working in a covers band, where nobody really cared what or how I sang as long as they could sing along with it and have a beer at the same time.

I wasn't disillusioned. I knew it would be tough to land a professional contract with a big show. But at 29, I had guts and determination on my side. I'd never been someone to sit back and 'wait' for opportunity. I was a hunter, thirsty for my big chance, and willing to fight for it. However, a decade of experience working in cabaret and covers bands seemed not to be enough to land me even a mid-range theatrical agent to represent me for the kinds of auditions and work I wanted. At the time, it felt like all the experience I had gained up until then had been void and trivial. My eyes had finally opened up to just how hard this new venture was going to be.

The journey continued as I spent months knocking on doors, only to be asked every time what 'professional' experience I'd had—since it seemed that none of the work I'd done in Adelaide was considered even moderately 'professional'. I felt, at 29, that I might have left my run a little too late. Perhaps I should have moved to Sydney earlier. I needed to land myself a musical theatre contract and that would give me the bargaining power to get myself an agent. Trouble was, without an agent you couldn't get an audition, and without an audition you couldn't get the job!

I started to feel desperate, but the hunter in me emerged. I took control of the situation and decided to bombard producers and production houses direct with my resume, hoping to score myself an audition as a freelance artist. From time to time, as the doubt crept back in, I started to think it would just be easier to go back home.

In our first year of moving to Sydney, I spread myself thinly across as many different areas as possible to get a foot in the door. I'd go from singing in our covers band on the weekends, to hiring musicians for corporate events, rehearsing new repertoires for the new acts we had put together, doing the invoicing and bookkeeping so that we all got paid. I took a daytime gig as MC at Sydney's Star City Casino to host their promotions and to give away money to the loyal gamblers. With all of this going on we were busy, but survived our first year in Sydney.

Shortly after turning 31, I finally got my first major break into the industry. It was in the chorus of the musical *The Producers*. My perseverance had paid off. I landed the audition myself by sending my resume and photo directly to the executive producer at the Gordon Frost Organisation. They were looking for five foot ten, blonde singing and dancing showgirls and I fitted the criteria perfectly. It was as simple as that. It didn't seem to matter what my experience had been beforehand. I fitted the mould physically, so the job was mine.

With that job offer in hand I became more saleable. I 'bought' myself an agent with the contract and took my first steps into the world of professional musical theatre. Finally achieving what I had always set out to do. In the back of my mind, the two years I dedicated to performing in this show was like bringing my life's dreams and goals to fruition, finally having something to show for the arduous years of the past. I had now earned my place in the industry working alongside theatre veterans such as Reg Livermore, Tom Burlinson and Bert Newton.

Getting into a musical was a major personal accomplishment, but coming up with the goods to sustain a professional performance eight times a week was another story altogether. Every moment on stage is tightly choreographed into what appears to the unsuspecting audience as an effortless combination of dialogue, singing, dance, moving scenery and impossibly quick costume changes. It was utterly exhausting, but I had to maintain my professional demeanour at all times. It must have worked as I was cast by the American producers as the understudy to one of the leading roles in the show—the Swedish secretary, Ulla.

The actress playing this role was a seasoned professional. She had long, flexible limbs, was impossibly tall and thin and had worked for years to earn her place in this show. It was her first major break and she deserved it and her shoes were big ones to fill. If she was ever to get sick and miss a show, I would be the 'unknown' stepping in to the limelight, trying to make sure the show ran as close to perfect as possible with as few as a couple of hours rehearsal time a week. It was a great opportunity for a first time showgirl like me. No longer a trained dancer, I was humbled at being selected. After all, I'd never been in a show before and had never even had an agent before now.

The producers must have thought I looked far more adept than I felt, because there was the point in the show when 'Ulla' had to back flip off a table and end up in a left leg split. All without using her hands to cushion her fall. It was a big ask of someone who could only just do the splits on the right leg. I couldn't even hold my own weight in a handstand, let alone flip backwards. But I wasn't letting on. I spent months upside down, doing handstands against a wall preparing myself for the moment I was called upon to step into the role and perform miracles. When the day finally came, I remember hearing my mum and Fez gasp from the audience as I flipped off that desk and landed in the splits with the loudest 'yeeha' I could muster. I'd done it! The show was a success. But everything comes at a price. In my enthusiasm to do the manoeuvre just right, I had fractured my left hip and was off the show for three months.

As they say in theatre: 'break a leg'. Just not literally I guess.

The Producers closed just after my 33rd birthday—and until this time I had never really thought about having a family. I guess I was too busy enjoying my career and proving something to myself. I never thought any of this could impact me later on down the track. But with the show over I had time to think. I started to wonder if I had been selfish. Had I put my own needs, hopes and desires before my fertility expiration date? I had always believed that one of the most selfish things a human being can do is take responsibility for another's life when they haven't yet conquered their own sense of self and purpose in this world. It made sense to me at the time. I would eventually become a mother when the time was right, when I was ready. It was a given.

Suddenly, in my new free time, my mind wandered far and wide and I was faced with the realisation I'd been off the pill for five years and hadn't fallen pregnant. Then the baby shower invites started to arrive. Of my 15 closest friends, nine were pregnant and expecting within six months of each other. I sighed as I said goodbye to the long ladies' lunches and the designer clothing which would soon make way for 10am brunches in the park, glasses of maison (alcohol-free wine, God forbid) and baby Dior.

I engrossed myself in sourcing impractical, original baby shower gifts and discovering the world of baby products that await expecting mothers. Watching others around me go through motherhood certainly made me curious to get started. I didn't want to be left behind. But five years? We weren't 'trying' to get pregnant, but it was puzzling why we hadn't accidentally got pregnant. The self doubt reared its ugly head again, and I started to worry.

CHAPTER 2

Why me?

> "M/cus . . . At the very moment I wrote that abbreviation, sex became science and charting was the new foreplay."

Year 1, November—
How would you like your eggs?

It's been a while since I first discussed the prospect of starting a family with Fez. He, like me, believes that it will happen when the time is right and that we shouldn't put too much emphasis on it. I've had a feeling, though, that things aren't going to be so easy. It's been niggling at me for some time. Surely our odds aren't good if I have been off the pill for five years. We're bound to have hit those magic fertile days 12, 14 or 16 within that time! I have started to do a bit of research on the internet and am discovering a wealth of information for aspiring parents: ovulation kits, thermometers, natural remedies, acupuncture, fertility pillows, folic acid, zinc. Just about anything and everything—including the most opportune days to have sex. As my desire for it to happen naturally and without aid is intensifying, I just feel so overwhelmed, and I don't know whose advice to take. Suddenly, having a baby is becoming a fully fledged production number. I just wanted something to come easy for a change.

I was never really any good at maths, but in my quest to increase our odds, I am now a master at graphs and charting. Last month I planned a weekend away with Fez which also 'happened' to fall on those magic fertile days of my cycle. I had it all mapped out. Spontaneity in my world is now a thing of the past—but I didn't want him to know that. We were to go away to the mountains for a few days of stress-free bliss. I planned it like a military operation. I chose a place called Lake Lyall in the Blue Mountains near Sydney as I had a romantic notion that we would fall pregnant and call our first son Lyall. On the way there we discussed prospective names for our children but there didn't seem to be many we could both agree on. I'm guessing this could prove to be a bone of contention in the future.

On the first night as we were settling in for a cosy evening by the fire, Fez found a graph that I had used to chart my basal temperatures. I explained to him the meaning behind the charting and how a woman can sometimes tell her most fertile period by temperature graphing and changes leading up to ovulation. I watched as he curiously peered closer at the chart to enquire about the meaning of the scribbled 'm/cus'. This is of course my discreet way of noting any changes in cervical mucus. At the very moment I wrote that abbreviation, sex became science and charting was the new foreplay.

Three days later, we were back at home and resumed life in the daily grind. I'd come away with some wonderful photos of our trip (just so we could show Lyall) as well as a urinary tract infection as a result of many vigorous late night baby-making sessions. I have always been a bit susceptible to these kinds of infections, and in retrospect I should have known I would get one, but there was a job to be done and I was going to do it no matter what.

Despite all our well planned efforts, my period arrived two weeks later and we were back to square one. Hey, I never really liked the name Lyall all that much anyway—and Fez hated it!

Many more months followed like this—mapping, charting, taking my temperature, and waiting, being disappointed. In those early days, I still had the energy to turn a negative into a positive. After all, that had always been my coping mechanism.

To increase our odds of getting pregnant, I tried standing on my head after sex, elevating the hips, herbal potions, cutting back on our beloved wine and cutting out artificial sugar and coffee. I told myself that there had to be something stopping us from falling pregnant. Of course by this time I had heard all the stories about how so and so had been trying for years and all it took was a holiday and a bit of R&R. Then there were Mike and Danni, the couple who put a couple of fertility dolls behind their bed head for a week to miraculously fall pregnant, as well as Jane and

Victor, the couple who never had sex and decided that a baby would strengthen their bond, so they went for it and on that particular night/day in the cycle/hour within the 24 hour window, fell pregnant. Stories like these were plentiful and sometimes offered brief hope, but more often than not caused more pain than promise.

It is time to do some further investigation. I am almost 34 and don't want to leave it any longer. I don't want to reach my forties and be left without a choice. I've researched everything I could find on the internet and considered every bit of advice from well-meaning friends, but I'm still not pregnant. I am getting exhausted failing month after month. Physically, it is tough but it is getting even harder emotionally. Sex for pleasure has become a distant memory and the schedule is beginning to take its toll. I am going to make an appointment to see my doctor for a referral to a fertility specialist. I need to clear my mind and work out what to do next. There is no point sitting around and waiting for things to happen anymore. We've gone beyond that now.

CHAPTER 3

Deciding it's out of your hands

> "I was amused when I was the only one asked if I exercised and followed a healthy diet. Clearly it should be just as important for the man in the relationship?"

Year 2, March—
Clinically infertile

It's taken me this long to come to terms with admitting that I'm defeated. Every time I start to process the magnitude of medical intervention required for our fertility woes, I am reminded that thousands of people fall pregnant naturally every month. I thought if I could just wait it out, I'd be another pregnancy statistic. I've been carrying around the referral to see a fertility specialist from my doctor for the last few months. I knew I'd have to make the phone call eventually, I was just hoping I wouldn't HAVE to. It would be easy to go about my life, ignoring this little piece of paper but I can't ignore the deep yearning I've developed of wanting to have a child of my own. I've asked myself 'why?', but at the end of the day it's just in me. I don't need a child to complete me, but I do need a child to feel complete. I want to watch them take their first breath of life and be that person to hold them close when nothing else can bring comfort. I want to marvel at their creation and I certainly want to hear the word 'mum'. I want to make fairy bread and let my child know that they are all that matters in this world. My world. They're all the simplest of things, and yet the hardest to achieve.

Up until recently, I only ever cared about my career and carving out a good future for myself and my husband. Now, as I think more about this life I've been given, I wonder if I'm missing some vital sign. My happiness has been so categorically determined by my career success. As soon as I tick a goal off the list, it's like I never really stop for a moment to really pat myself on the back. Instead, I spend my energy striving for the next big leap in what often seems like an unattainable feat. It's like a drug. I go for an audition, get a job, feel good about myself for a few hours and then come crashing back down to earth. Ultimately who really cares if I am the voice behind a radio campaign you hear as you're driving to work in the morning? Who cares if I sing the national anthem for a televised audience at the football? Who cares if my name is in the programme of a glossy musical theatre production, barely recognisable, hidden behind elaborate sets, fancy costumes and heavy stage makeup? It is all so forgettable and you're always only as good as your last job. It takes so much energy to keep striving for bigger and better things, not to mention picking yourself up after the frequent knockbacks. It's a crazy profession and the industry's flooded with younger, better looking and more talented people wherever I turn. Competing takes effort. Effort that is valuable. Effort that I want to spend elsewhere, making a difference and contributing to this world. I'm tired of spending my whole life on a diet and feeling the pressure to line up for the latest cosmetic treatment. Maybe I'm already too old.

Today is the first of many baby steps taken in our pursuit of 'assisted' parenthood. This afternoon we have our first appointment with a fertility specialist. He will give us advice on treatment options and dissect our fertility history. I honestly never thought we would get to this stage and a dark cloud looms over me. What will we be asked? Will we have to admit that sex has perhaps not been happening as frequently lately, as potentially it should be? Will we lie to save face? Do we say we have been trying for a year, or do we just count the months that we have really 'gone for it'? We have decided I will answer the more personal questions and we'll approach the others with caution. I am not ready for any self analysis or heaven knows, marital counselling.

Later that day

We met with a well-respected fertility specialist at 2 pm. He came highly recommended from a girlfriend. There is some comfort in that. As Fez and I took a seat in the swanky waiting room, I was quietly advised to empty my bladder as the doctor may like to do an internal examination right there and then. My face drained. I usually have to psyche myself up two months in advance just to get a pap smear! I only kept the appointment because I had exhausted all plausible excuses and am too embarrassed to re-schedule. (I have a problem getting massages too.)

Note to self: Book in with a psychiatrist to get my head examined once I have paid off this appointment!

On that note, it is certainly not going to be a cheap exercise. We have private health cover but, as I am discovering, the things you need most are almost always not covered. It was around $200 just for today's initial appointment and I get the impression these might go on for months, not to mention the tests and procedures that we now have to do.

As we were waiting to be seen by the doctor, my mind was thinking back to what undies I had put on today. I had heart palpitations when I realised it had been a few days since I'd gotten the old razor out. I suddenly forgot all about the real reasons why we were here and started visualising the region down below. Fez grabbed himself a copy of the latest Who magazine and kept himself amused, unaware of my inner turmoil.

Then: 'Mr and Mrs Krizak. This way please.'

I gingerly left my seat and followed the receptionist into Dr Fertility's office. I felt something trickle down my leg. 'Please let it be sweat,' I thought. We took a seat and proceeded to meet our doctor. He had an unusual Australian accent and was very friendly indeed. I began to relax and feel like

I was having a chat with a good mate. All small talk to start with, general chit chat and patient details. Then the doctor pulled out a folder with some paperwork that resembled a census form.

My eyes scanned the questions, processing whatever I could while reading upside down. The questions seemed fairly straight forward and he assured us they were critical in building a patient's health profile. I was amused when I was the only one asked if I exercised and followed a healthy diet. Clearly it was just as important for the man in the relationship? This was the first major inconsistency as the doctor's voice started to resonate in my ear.

'Mrs. Krizak, unfortunately it is all about your eggs,' Dr Fertility said matter of factly. 'If Fez is fine in the sperm department, then it's all down to you.'

The questions varied from whether either of us had 'obtained a pregnancy' before, details about any recreational drug use, alcohol consumption. Hold on a minute, binge drinking? Ah no, maybe four to five glasses of wine a week? Uh hum. Moistness in the groin area again. Thank God the attention turned to Fez.

'Alcohol consumption Mr Krizak?'

'Binge drinker,' Fez replied, without a moment's hesitation.

Was he proud of this or something? I don't know what has gotten into him. I gripped the arm of his chair and looked at him in horror. The doctor smirked and replied with some smart-arsed comment that stereotypically related to a rock and roll lifestyle. In the midst of my embarrassment, Fez was given a gentle reminder that alcohol in moderation is always best for both would-be parents when trying to conceive. (Let me tell you, there was so much more we needed to get checked out before we would be giving that serious attention).

Dr Fertility asked me to take a seat on the bed next to his office table. It was all a bit too 'casting couch' for my liking. Who has a bed next to their office desk? This only happens in the movies when the young starlets come in for an 'audition' and are asked to display more than their 'acting' talents. Nevertheless, I complied, and took my place on the sterile, white-sheeted bed. Dr Fertility asked me to remove my underwear. This was getting uncomfortable. We'd only just met. I took myself to that 'out of body' place, removed my jeans and underwear and placed one of the bed sheets over my lower half. That's when Dr Fertility introduced me to the 'follicle wand'. He said it would feel like a pap smear and could determine the amount of follicles present on each ovary. This would give him an insight into how my ovaries looked and whether there was anything abnormal about their appearance. As he worked, he rattled off the numbers nine and seven—nine on the right, seven on the left. It was a decent number of follicles apparently. Still, he couldn't tell the quality of the eggs inside the ovaries. Quality not quantity as the saying goes. The whole procedure was over in five minutes and Dr Fertility was back at his desk before I could pull up my pants. This was all as normal to him as brushing his teeth in the morning. I guess I'd better get myself familiar with the embarrassment too if we are to get some answers. Let the journey begin.

Half an hour later, we were on our way home with Dr Fertility's last words still ringing in our heads:

"Just remember, you're not that ancient and we should be able to achieve success through IVF."

So, I'm 'not that ancient'. Just how ancient is 'ancient'? (Ironically the clinic also offers botox injections for those feeling a little more than 'not that ancient'. Maybe I'll need some of that later for the frown lines I am already acquiring from only one appointment).

We got home and my first port of call was to check to see what had been running down my leg earlier. There was nothing there. It must have been just sweat after all. Phew.

CHAPTER 4

After your first visit, what's next?

"There's almost always a solution to every problem. It's finding the problem that takes time."

Year 2, April—
Tests, trials and testes

One of the first things we are asked to do is to get our blood tested, so all the routine checks could be done and any STDs ruled out. It was imperative that I had mine done mid-cycle so that all the hormone levels could be checked to see if I am actually ovulating. Fez was also asked to book himself in for a 'semen analysis'. At our most recent appointment he was given a jar to collect the sample in, and then told to get it back to the clinic within the hour. The semen sample had to be kept at body temperature until we delivered it to the clinic, and the best place for that, ironically, was tucked securely between my legs or in my cleavage. You don't need a grand imagination to gather how a man comes up with a semen sample, so I'll leave it at that. However, I do hear the fancier clinics come equipped with discreet rooms that include plasma TV's with sophisticated 'adult films' and a strategically placed box of disinfectant wipes next to the remote control. Without delving into too much detail and risking my marriage completely, the sample was produced and delivered for testing along with our 'bloods'.

In these past few weeks, since our first appointment I have had a total of four blood tests done. I have had so many vials of blood taken, I am hoping that the answer will lie in a test tube somewhere so at least we may soon know what was exactly wrong with us and rectify the problem. I always get my period on day 28, so naturally I am presuming I am ovulating OK.

Perhaps the problem is with Fez. You hear about that a lot. It is not uncommon for the man to be producing inadequate sperm. Sperm that don't swim, sperm that are mostly dead, or sperm that clump together. We'd have to wait and see what the results of Fez's sperm analysis were. I've been reading about a procedure called ICSI which is helpful to couples trying to conceive with inadequate sperm. It's where one single sperm is selected and injected into the egg itself, giving the couple the best possible chance of success. If it came down to that, we would look into this procedure for sure. I'm beginning to learn so much more about the benefits of science and research. There's almost always a solution to every problem. It's finding the problem that takes the time.

Year 2, Mid-April

The phone hasn't rung since the testing, so I am confident that nothing serious has been detected. The visits to the specialist are getting easier. I've noticed all types of people coming and going. Some older, some quite young. Some with their partners, others with their mothers holding their hand.

I must admit I am really missing my mum. Because our families live in Adelaide, to include them in all of this would only make for unease on their behalf. I mentioned to my mum and a few close friends that we were having some investigation done into why we couldn't conceive but I downplayed the most of it, which kept the intrusive questioning at bay. We have decided to go this alone for the time being, and deal with whatever is about to be thrust upon us. Pity was one thing I certainly did not want.

We took our seats in our doctor's office again today, waiting with baited breath as he retrieved the combination of lab results and mused over our paperwork. I took a minute to have a look at all the photos of babies around the room. All of them there because of others like us who sat in these chairs and hoped for a miracle. I wonder if our child will ever make the walls of his office. The silence was broken by the sound of Dr Fertility's pen ticking items off our list and jotting down some kind of medical jargon that accompanies each test. I sat on the edge of my chair as he peered over the top of his glasses at our results on the paper. No sweat trickling down my leg—good!

'STDs—nil, Rubella vaccination—still immune, Blood types—compatible, Sperm—good quantity, normal. Eggs—Ovulation occurring, hormones evident and normal. Slight age deterioration, to be expected. Nothing abnormal. Verdict—9 percent chance of conceiving naturally.'

Hang on a minute. I felt optimistic. Nothing negative had been found, so we should be OK and able to conceive naturally. It's just a timing thing surely? So why the 9 percent? That verdict really knocked me for six. I was still getting over my initial shock, when I asked the doc why the chances of us conceiving naturally were so low. He told us that even an average, healthy couple under 25 has only a 20-25 percent chance of conceiving in any given month and cycle. Why on earth do we worry ourselves so much when we're younger and go on the pill! I had no idea the odds were so low to get pregnant, yet people seem to achieve it so effortlessly and have done so for thousands of years. Christ, we have a nine percent chance, not 20-25 percent. Is the difference just because I'm 'not that ancient'? Nine percent are not the greatest odds. So because I have been off the pill for five or so years, I am technically 'infertile'. Basically, if it hasn't happened by now it is never going to. To make matters worse, we are one of the 30 percent of all 'infertile' couples that are inconclusive, meaning there isn't a medical explanation as to why. We've come a full circle. Infertile until proven otherwise.

The next step to take is a process of elimination tests. We are told that there are many options available to us, but we first have to decide just how far we want to delve into the medical reasons as to why we can't fall pregnant.

Year 2, Late April—
Anyone for chicken?

Our next scheduled appointment was basically to discuss our options and the extent of intrusive testing that we were prepared to undergo. It is decision time and getting increasingly harder for me to stay focused on the long-term goal.

I decided that a hysterosalpingogram (HSG) would make the most sense in determining if there was anything biologically wrong with me. I was told that it would be intrusive but no more discomfort than your average pap smear. Grimace. A HSG involves having a catheter inserted into the vagina and up through the cervix, where a radioactive dye can then be sent up through the tube to see if the fallopian tubes are clear and open. An x-ray machine simultaneously shows the effects on a nearby monitor. This procedure is designed to rule out any blockages in the fallopian tubes which could prevent the sperm getting to the ovaries.

I arrived at the clinic and was met by a nurse who gave me a gown to change into and instructed me to remove my underwear. I was then ushered into a small room where I was placed on a bed that resembled something out of a dental clinic. I am used to spotlights in my profession but this was one mighty big spotlight in all the wrong places. I took a deep breath as the doctor prepared me for what was about to eventuate. He said it should only take a few minutes and that I might experience some minor discomfort as the dye was released. There was also a chance that I could have an allergic reaction to the dye but that only happened in an extreme minority of cases. He told me that

27

sometimes the procedure itself dislodges any obstructions in the fallopian tubes and a few women have been known to fall pregnant following it. I felt optimistic.

'Keep very still for me Debora and we'll take a photo at various stages of the procedure so we can determine what is going on', said Dr Fertility.

I think he sensed my uneasiness. I started to think about his job. How does a man do this day after day, staring at the female anatomy? What would their sex lives be like? Surely they would have seen some sights to put them off for life?

I was distracted from my train of thought when he started to tell the Nurse about the Portuguese chicken shop he had stumbled upon in Petersham over the weekend. Chicken? Chicken? Is that what my private parts reminded him of or was he just so de-sensitised to all of this that he could just switch off and talk about chicken? Surely all this tricky work wasn't making him hungry? Which comes first the chicken or the egg? By then, I had turned bright red. I hoped I wasn't having an allergic reaction.

As promised, it was, in fact, all over in a few minutes and the nurse kindly gave me a sanitary pad to place under me so that I could catch the leaking dye when I stood up. 'Just how am I supposed to do this discreetly?' I wondered, succeeding in rolling myself off the bed in a manoeuvre that only an Olympic gymnast could appreciate. I got myself changed and was soon back to some semblance of my dignified self. The procedure had been a success and no blockages were discovered, which once again eliminated another factor and left me high (but not so dry) as to what the problem might be.

On the way out, I was given a pile of paperwork to take home and read. The next step after a HSG is to opt for a combined hysteroscopy and a laparoscopy. I was told that this procedure involves an operation whereby a small tube fitted with a camera is inserted into the abdomen, which can identify any signs of scar tissue within the uterus and fallopian tubes. This could be one of my potential problems. If the egg can't travel down the tubes to meet up with the sperm, then no baby. Scarring can occur as a result of a previous operation. But I haven't had any 'previous operations' so that's not a consideration for me. In some cases endometriosis can be lasered off at the time of the operation, as well as any cysts that may have been found on the ovaries. I found another brochure that informed me that cysts can also hinder egg release.

The combined hysteroscopy and a laparoscopy is an actual operation and I am not quite as open to going under the knife as I am to having my ovaries probed in my quest to eliminate infertility factors. I would happily do everything in my power to have a baby, but as there is never any guarantee that this will happen, I feel that having an operation to 'see' if anything is wrong, compromises my own life as well as the potential to give life down the track. If nothing else, at least my husband has me and I have him. It isn't our ideal scenario but it will be better than chancing it on an operating table.

There I go again, letting random thoughts run away with me. I often catch myself dramatising every situation, just as I do in my day-to-day life as a performer. But if it isn't broken, don't fix it, right? Technically, I am not broken—a little fractured and uneasy maybe but, in essence, I still have faith in my reproductive organs. I liken this faith to my ability to keep going in the face of adversity—after suffering knockback after knockback in my career, still having enough self belief that I will reach the end goal, without compromising myself to get there.

Thankfully Dr Fertility assured us that, in the long run, if anything is wrong internally, then an IVF procedure will bypass it altogether and we can achieve the same desired result without having to have further operations.

It seems like a lifetime of work needs to be done before Fez and I can reach our goal of having a baby. This is feeling like every other aspect of my life—tests (auditions), waiting for results (call backs) and uncertainty. I was already tired of that life and ready to put that chapter behind me. But now I am facing the same hurdles in my reproductive life. I am starting to realise you can't escape your destiny, and this journey set before me isn't going to be an easy one on any account.

Year 2, Mid-May—
Sometimes life doesn't give us a choice

I have taken a few weeks off since my last entry trying to gather my thoughts and contemplate the reality of becoming an IVF patient. When can we start? Can we afford it? How much will it cost exactly? How many disappointments will we have to go through before we are successful? And even then, is it worth it when the miscarriage rate is considerably higher than a natural pregnancy?

I am back on the internet (of course). Can Fez and I cope with this? I heard somewhere that one in three couples have an extremely hard time dealing with the emotional turmoil and stress that IVF brings. Some people even compare the stress levels of a couple going through IVF to having the same impact as someone suffering from a major terminal illness.

What if the synthetic hormones turn me into a psychopath? Would Fez abandon me? We've always been such a rational, clear-thinking couple. Will my body suffer? I'm worried about looking pregnant without actually being pregnant and being the subject of everyone's suspicions (but without a certain reward). The sheer volume of fluid in the ovaries could make me look at least three months pregnant. How will I explain the weight gain to clients? Let's just say I am petrified—about everything.

Fez is my eternal optimist, my rock. He is used to picking me up out of the depths of despair. He has always been there when I have been close to my dream role, only to find out I had been pipped at the post by someone else. I have had to become good at disguising my disappointment so I can soldier on with the next audition or prospect that presents itself. Thank God for Fez.

Men like to fix things—things around the house, cars, in fact anything that is repairable. When it comes to women, men like to be able to fix our emotions and make everything alright again and they do this with optimism. I know I am generalising here, but it can be a huge hurdle for a man when he can't make things 'right'. Subsequently when he can't control an outcome he will try to find the light at the end of it all and assure us that everything will be on track again soon. Men seem to spend more time thinking about the 'now' and a lot less about the 'what ifs' of the future.

Fez hates to see me upset. After all, he married a strong, independent woman. One that fights in the face of adversity and rises to a challenge. I try to portray dignity and strength, even when things are falling apart around me. But what he and others don't see is the late night silent sobbing into my pillow. It's my way of releasing when I just can't hold the fort up any longer.

Sometimes wanting something so desperately means that letting go becomes part of a grieving process and that takes time. We only ever read about the people who achieve great things in life. The people who win the lottery, those who miraculously achieve their goals by luck, or discover their passion by some chance encounter. We don't hear about the rest of us who struggle day to day, working hard to earn a living, having let our dreams and desires go, through no fault of our own. We never celebrate the battlers. The universe doesn't 'open up for them', nor do they receive a helping hand from the 'Gods above'. They simply have to give up and spend the rest of their lives completely aware that their dreams are just a fantasy that will never come to fruition. Yet we're told it's good to dream. Don't give up on your dreams. It's good to live like those poor kids on TV talent shows every year who torment themselves (and us) by 'following their dreams'. I wonder how they feel when they end up on the 'best of the worst' segment for our viewing pleasure. I wonder if they think it was worth it? When does a parent squash a child's dream when it is blatantly obvious that their offspring is not cut out for their chosen profession? What would I do in those circumstances?

Where am I going with all of this? I'm not entirely sure. When obstacles come up in life it makes you look at things philosophically. I've had plenty of time to ponder about the 'what ifs'. I am scared of what the future might bring but somewhere in the back of my mind, I know the old Deb still exists. There is a glimmer of hope and aspiration. I do still believe in the fairytale ending and probably will until the day I die. I believe the universe will come through for us. I'm not ready to let go just yet.

Year 2, Late May—
Career versus Family

Fez and I have agreed to take six months off after deciding to proceed with IVF. There are a number of reasons for our decision. The first being I have just scored a minor role in the Australian debut of Titanic: A New Musical, playing the part of a French millionaire passenger, Madame Aubert. I only have three lines but it is a step up from being a sequin-clad showgirl in The Producers. I am actually being recognised as an established singer/actor. It is a short season and means I don't have to put too much on hold to participate. It came along very easily. I did very little preparation for my audition and was still deliberating as to whether I would even turn up, right up until the night before. Being offered this job is a stroke of luck and a welcome relief.

I discussed putting IVF off for those six months between appointments with the doc. Financially it will be better to start at the beginning of the year due to the Medicare rebate, which will enable us to claim back up to 80% of our out of pocket expenses. This will also coincide with the end of my Titanic contract. The prospect of starting afresh in the new year is really appealing. In the meantime, we can have six months to continue trying to conceive naturally. Maybe we will be one of those couples—and defy our 9 percent medical odds.

Our next appointment with Dr Fertility is November 22.

CHAPTER 5

I'll try anything

"28 days can be a long time when you are trying for a baby. Each month was an excruciating wait."

During the six months that followed I went back and re-researched everything I possibly could on the internet to enhance our nine per cent chance of achieving a pregnancy. I purchased fertility vitamins, ovulation thermometers, examined changes in cervical mucus and hung upside down at every possible post-coital opportunity. It became a hobby and an interest. It consumed my every waking minute. I found a local Chinese herbalist who also specialised in acupuncture and natural fertility treatment. I was given a six month course of the most disgusting, vile-tasting herbs that I was instructed to boil up and drink twice a day—morning and night—with the aim of regulating my hormones and promoting fertility. The end product looked like I'd taken a cup of the dirtiest water I could find and, once boiled, I had to drink every last drop, all whilst holding my nose to protect my tastebuds from the assault of the putrid taste. I tried to convince myself that this stuff was actually beneficial to me. Taking the herbs in conjunction with regular acupuncture sessions was a double whammy. As my Chinese doctor placed fine needles all over my 'fertility' points, I was challenged to take myself off to a place of pure relaxation and positive thoughts. Unfortunately, the only thought I could muster was when my next lot of dirty water was due. I can't say it did much for my state of mind.

For Fez, it was sex on tap. Not just at ovulation time (we found that unreliable) but all month round—just to make sure we covered every possible window. For me, it was as mandatory as writing the daily shopping list. My body didn't even get the chance to become aroused. My mind had completely taken over. There was a job to be done and under the circumstances, the quicker it could be done, the better. My body was simply a piece of machinery. I was completely detached from the whole sexual experience. It was no more meaningful to me than going for a daily blood test. It was all part of the process. I had completely succumbed to the ritual.

I meticulously planned our most fertile days. As each monthly period approached, I would get excited and found myself reviewing all my hard work researching online, spending hours analysing my diary to make sure we had covered all windows of opportunity. We gave it our best shot and were the most committed we had ever been. Fez said he felt like an event planner which quite honestly summed things up perfectly.

A couple of months passed without results and with it came the monthly sinking feeling once my period arrived. I was like clockwork. Every 28 days to the dotted 'P' in the diary. It felt like there was still time and we felt we could still experiment with a few different timing options. One month we would aim for the earlier part of the cycle, another month we would try the later half. It was like a game of 'join the dots'.

Ovulation kits gave me another tool to draw on. I bought a test that could detect a women's fertile window from a swab of saliva examined under a lipstick sized magnifying glass. Even I marvelled as the microscope showed up a fern like pattern just as the instructions stated when a woman was ovulating. This was the ideal time to make a baby according to the test. It was a nifty little gadget and I was hoping this would be the secret weapon in our quest to fall pregnant naturally. I'd look obsessively for the "ferns" every single day and once the pattern emerged, I'd make extra effort to make love more than once on that particular day. Then it was up to the gods . . . oh and the herbs, needles and ferns. 28 days can be a very long time when you are trying for a baby. Each month was an excruciating wait.

Year 2, Late July—
DES Daughter

Today I received a call from my mother in Adelaide. She had been to the doctor for her annual check up and had picked up a magazine in the doctor's waiting room. She sounded panicked on the phone.

"Deb, do you remember me telling you how I started miscarrying when I was pregnant with you at nine weeks?"

"Vaguely mum, but you elevated your legs and called the night doctor and everything was normal right?"

"Well I'm not sure if I told you or not, but that night the doctor gave me an injection and some tablets to take to prevent any further bleeding . . . I only took one of the tablets and threw the rest away . . . But I have just read an article in the doctor's surgery about a condition in the daughters of mothers who were prescribed the drug DES to prevent miscarriages in the 70s. It causes infertility and abnormalities of the female reproductive organs."

My heart skipped a beat.

"I'm not sure what the drug was that I was prescribed Deb, but I have kept this article and will send it off to you so you can talk it over with your specialist."

"OK mum, I'm sure it's nothing to worry about but I'll call my specialist and mention it to him all the same."

"Deb, I hope I haven't done anything to cause any of this trouble you have been having. I couldn't live with myself if I was the cause of all this. Please go and get it all checked out for me."

I reassured mum that it would be OK, hung up and went straight to the internet and tried to find out whatever I could about DES daughters. She was right in saying that it causes infertility in some women who were subjected to this drug while in their mother's womb. Apparently it is an ongoing case study and one that will not be conclusive as to what the effects of the drugs are until most daughters are in their reproductive years. Prior to this, most young women would not even know that they had been subjected to such a drug.

DES stands for Diethylstilbestrol. It can cause deformities in the uterus of an unborn female child. The main indicator is a T-shaped uterus which is often the first sign of exposure to the drug. It is also becoming evident that rare types of vaginal and cervical cancers are developing as a result of exposure.

As most of these daughters were born in the 70s, the full extent of the impact on them will not be realised until the cancers start developing and it gets traced back to DES.

I called Dr Fertility and mentioned the DES concern and he assured me that my HSG scan would have shown up any deformities in the uterus and he is confident that I am clear of the drug. Still, I was just amazed how quickly and easily he could dismiss this possibly vital piece of information. He once again reiterated that IVF would bypass any issues like this. I am beginning to feel like I am just another name in Dr Fertility's little black cheque book. This clinic's protocol appears to set aside the potential fertility issues at hand and cut straight to the chase of producing a baby with science. There's a formula for that. No one seemed to know any other way to treat my unexplained infertility. I hope I fit into the text book formula.

Year 2, August—
Calm before the storm

Of course there isn't any scientific proof that I haven't been subjected to DES, but as I don't have any of the obvious signs or symptoms, I am happy to declare myself unaffected. The only reminder is the familiar failing to fall pregnant each month. No one seems too perturbed, except mum of course. But then, that's what mothers do. Worry (apparently).

We still have three months of trying to conceive naturally before our next specialist appointment. This is it. The day we will officially admit defeat and lock in our first date with IVF in the New Year. It doesn't seem real that we are even considering it. This won't happen to us. We will make it on our own. Get over the line. Be one of the 'lucky' ones.

Year 2, September

Rehearsals for my new show Titanic: A New Musical had started. I was nervous and excited to meet the cast, and couldn't wait to commence work on what is my new life's focus for the next few months. At least it is going to take my mind off our conception issues and make me feel relatively normal again. I'm excited to be working on a musical again. It's great to have something new to talk about (and to think about for that matter).

I'm pretty sure my friends are tired of my conception trials and tribulations, especially when pregnancy came so easy to all of them. It is definitely a shock to the system. I still have a few trusted older friends who are yet to procreate and seem blissfully unaware of their own impending ovarian demise. It is comforting to know that I am not the only one left standing. However the one tiny difference is that they are on the pill and not trying for a family yet. They still have things they want to get done before embarking on that journey. Thank God for them. Spending time with them temporarily diverts my thoughts and makes me feel alive again. There isn't any baby talk, we can catch up at a moment's notice and the topic of conversation is usually centred around the latest handbag accessory or gossip tabloid. Refreshing.

Every now and then, I open up about my struggle to conceive, but I guess most of my friends just think we are unlucky. I don't think any of them really give much thought to the fact that infertility isn't just a one-off incident that is only happening to me. There is no point in me preaching to others and advising them to get a move on with their own conception journey, especially as I have so many friends over 35 who fell pregnant almost immediately. No-one has reason to think they should have any trouble. I am the freak. People always think it will still just happen when they least expect it. That's the advice I hear the most. We are simply trying too hard. I have even been told to get myself a Golden Retriever puppy to bring out my maternal urges. This will apparently make me more fertile. It's hard not to grab these people round the neck and shake them. They think our lack of baby equates to a lack of REALLY wanting a child. According to this group of people, I subconsciously don't want a family. Even my family doctor in Adelaide told my mum this. He said I am most likely 'blocking' my husband's sperm (whatever THAT means) because I am too concerned I would become pregnant and forever lose my 'figure'. Great. Another thing I have to reassure my poor mother about. (Ironically, I've never thought of myself as having a particularly 'spoilable' figure. But I digress . . .)

Year 2, October—
All creatures great and small

I have been immersing myself in my work. Titanic rehearsals run for six days a week from ten in the morning until six at night (the closest hours I've ever had to a real job!) Rehearsals are always a time of uncertainty and pressure. Pressure to remember every song, cue and direction. Pressure to be everything the producers were hoping you'd be from the initial audition. And then there is the pressure for the show to surpass the critics' expectations and have a long, successful run in the theatre where the producers' investments all pay off. No pressure, really.

It's always awkward walking into a new job and meeting 50 unfamiliar faces for the first time. The first week is usually strained but most of us start to bond fairly quickly and work out who are the show-offs, and who are the cast drunks. There's a real hierarchy system in theatre. You can usually determine how important you are by whether the producer makes an actual effort to come over and shake your hand or kiss you on the cheek. If you're not a leading player, you take your seat somewhere towards the back and go mostly unrecognised. Of course there are always those few people who will impose their humour and personality onto everyone, striving to get noticed amongst the crowd.

Good for them, but I'm not interested in that kind of carry on. It bores me and takes up too much energy.

I am slowly getting myself back into the mindset of doing eight shows a week. Welcome to musical theatre—there's not much of a life outside of it. Any time off you get is spent either partying or sleeping. It's quite a mundane experience and yet some people love it so much they go from show to show, year after year, locking themselves into two-year contracts, where they perform the same show in exactly the same way, at the same time, every night and day. (A lot like my sex life I guess. But there I go, digressing again!)

This month's baby making was a write-off. Fez is ill and is in no mood for my pre-ovulatory reminders about our ticking fertility clock. We also experience one of the biggest tragedies in our baby-obsessed lives—the loss of our beloved pet budgie Doofus.

Doofus was affectionately known as our 'special child'. He couldn't fly and relied on us to pick him up off the floor and take him to his chosen destinations. He had his own unique way of communicating with us and was such a happy little bird. We also have a cockatiel named Jezzabelle, and Doofus' sole purpose for living was to woo this larger female bird and hope that one day she would let him mate her. It was just gorgeous to watch. He never gave up.

We had Doofus for five years and he was our first Sydney-bred budgie. As his age progressed and his health deteriorated, we did our best to make him comfortable and give him the best quality of life. Fez took a particular liking to him and was responsible for his treatment and making sure Doofus didn't overeat. (Domestic birds have a habit of not knowing when to stop eating!!)

Sadly, though, Doofus died in tragic circumstances and (out of respect for Fez) I am not going to retell exactly how he met his death. Suffice it to say that Fez is inconsolable and I am scared to leave him alone with his grief. So I cancelled my work for today and we dedicate ourselves to laying our little Doof Doof to rest in the park across the road. Not many people understand the magnitude at which one can love a bird and fail to see how birds can compare to more conventional pets like dogs and cats, but believe me they do! I'd never thought of our love for Doofus as being anything out of the norm. It wasn't until the deep devastation kicked in that we both realised there was a lot more to this situation than just losing a pet. We need something to nurture. Nurturing came naturally with Doofus. We have deferred all of our yearnings for a baby onto this poor little bird and in the end it was probably our love that killed him over anything else. Yes, we overfed him, yes, we let him chew on potentially toxic objects around the house and yes, we littered his cage with as many brain stimulating, budgie loving toys as we could find. He was just another blue and white budgie but the sadness was magnificently overwhelming. RIP Doofy. Know that you were loved—whatever the reason.

I've heard it said that when people experience a natural disaster and are faced with tragedy and death, the result is quite often a spike in the population. Many people deal with the situation by doing what comes naturally, procreating. Somehow it eases the pain and in some way can divert people's attention from the mass disaster. I can understand this human defence.

One of my closest girlfriends called today and told me that perhaps Doofus was gone to make way for another little angel to come into our lives—I hope she is right and, in a way, I feel comforted by the thought.

Year 2, Friday 6 October—
Light at the end of the tunnel

Today they informed us that Titanic may go on tour and we have been asked to consider a tour in the first four months of the new year. The cast was ecstatic. It means four months of not having to worry about where the next pay cheque is coming from. But while they rejoiced in the offer, I turned it down. I need to be free in January for our IVF treatment. Hopefully it won't come down to that, but even if I did fall pregnant naturally in the next few months, I still wouldn't be able to tour. I'm already fantasising about who I would break the baby news to first. Mum for sure.

Actually, right now there are even greater things occupying my mind. My period is three days late and I'm feeling butterflies in my tummy. Could this be it? I knew the Gods would come through for me eventually. Its perfect timing. Mum arrives for a visit in a few days and it would make for a wonderful surprise to have her here when I break the news. Things are actually looking up and I'm feeling optimistic. I've made a pact with myself, if I haven't got my period by Sunday, I'll take a test in the morning and confirm it. That

45

also happens to be the day I pick mum up from the airport. I've never been late past 30 days and today is day 31.

Year 2, Saturday 7 October, 5 pm—
A Hallmark moment

It's early Saturday evening and all I can think about is those two pink lines. I feel myself succumbing to the thought of taking the pregnancy test tonight. I have it all mapped out it my mind. I won't tell Fez. I will do it on the quiet. Of course, if the result is negative I will be an emotional wreck after all this built-up excitement of the past few days and I'll have to talk to him straight away. I have pictured all the events as they will unfold in my mind like a movie. I haven't told Fez my period is late as I want to make it into a spectacular affair. God knows we have waited long enough for this moment, trying to be genuinely ecstatic about all our friends' triumphant pregnancies, willingly attending showers and braving the endless questions about our own fertility. Now it feels like it's our time to share the good news.

In preparation for my jubilant announcement, I went out shopping this morning and found myself drawn into a fancy card shop where the kind of cards they sell make me bawl my eyes out. I gravitated towards the baby section and glanced at all the 'congratulations' cards. I pictured how I would assemble all our cards in a fancy baby arrival scrap book! It brought a smile to my face and for a moment I forgot about the looming pregnancy test. Prolonging the test allows me to live in a state of hopeful bliss and not knowing offers more comfort to me than getting a negative result.

Back to the cards. My eyes were fixed on a card with the words "daddy" peering out at me. I suddenly had another romantic notion. What if I take Fez out to breakfast tomorrow morning and casually pass him this card that reads: "Congratulations daddy". Wouldn't that be spectacular? I wouldn't say a word and would wait for his look of bewilderment to subside before jumping up to embrace him. I didn't think for a moment that I was jumping the gun, so I purchased the card. I had convinced myself that I was pregnant and I was making it my little secret. Butterflies in the tummy again. I leave the card shop skipping all the hallmark tear jerkers and, as I made my way home, I made one final stop to the public toilets to re-affirm my pregnancy hopes. Still no period. I had at least gone a whole hour without checking. Not long to go before I will know for sure.

Should I test or should I not? I promised myself I'd wait until Sunday. One hour to go until I have to leave for work. If I want total privacy the best option for me would be to take it at work. If I get there early enough I will have the whole dressing room to myself. Perfect.

Year 2, Saturday 7 October, 7 pm—
Two Pink Lines

I walked to work fantasising about the new season's fashions and how the baby doll style would finally be flattering on me. I smiled at families enjoying their tea overlooking Darling Harbour and the tourists bustling about the city. Sydney really is a breathtaking city.

Rehearsals moved to the theatre a couple of days ago and I arrived with sweaty palms and a wiry pulse. This was it. No more delaying. I signed on to the cast arrival sheet and made my way down the stairs to my dressing room. There was no sign of life and the building was devoid of the usual wailing of fellow cast mates doing their warm up routines. It was dark and smelled of hairspray. I switched on the lights, inspected my complexion in the Hollywood mirrors and proceeded to the bathroom.

I pulled out the pregnancy kit that I had carefully selected for its high accuracy and scrutinised the instructions. It's not like I had never done one of these before, but I had to alleviate all possibilities of getting a false result by abiding by the packet instructions. They were like the bible to me. Hold the stick downwards, pee on it directly for exactly five seconds, then lay it on a flat surface and wait no longer than three minutes to determine the result. Heart palpitations. I wished Fez was there.

Two minutes passed, nothing. Just one bold pink line. The kind of line I have become accustomed to. Three minutes. Still only one line in the control window. Palpitations turned to perspiration. How could this be? I was almost six days overdue. It had to be wrong! As I sat staring at that little stick, my dreams shattered and my hopes dissolved. How I wished so desperately that just one of those tests would show TWO pink lines. If I stared at the strip long enough I could maybe fool myself into thinking a second pink line was appearing but after blinking a few times, the truth was evident. Would I ever be that lucky? I put the cap back on the test and hid it in with my makeup bag.

I can't help asking myself over and over again if these tests actually work. Maybe a blood test is the only reliable way to tell. Who am I kidding? The test was negative and I hadn't even shared these few days of hope with Fez. I feel as if I have cheated him that brief joy. I sat on the toilet seat and tears streamed down my face. Later, during the show's dress rehearsal, I didn't cry in the lifeboat scene, I sobbed, which earned me a tight squeeze from Madame Cardoza in the lifeboat seat next to me. My mind tricked me into thinking I was pregnant. I thought all along if you truly believed in something, then it would materialise. I'd even fooled myself.

CHAPTER 6

Dealing with Disappointment

"Tonight I just imagined singing to a child I should have had in my twenties. I'm singing about missed opportunity and unrealized dreams and the tears just flowed."

Year 2, Sunday 8 October—
Picking up the pieces

Today is Sunday. I drove to the airport to pick up my mum. The disappointment still weighing me down and the tears still fresh on my cheeks. I knew that seeing mum would make me even more emotional. I had thought a lot about my folks in the past year. My problems with fertility somehow make me feel like I am letting them down and depriving them of their rightful duties as grandparents. This is what chokes me up the most. Thankfully, they have recently been blessed with their first grandchild, a boy named Felix and the son of my eldest brother, Steve. He was such a joy and the few times I have seen him have filled me with pride. He is the most gorgeous child I had ever seen, and he isn't even mine. Thank God for him. Seeing my parents hold him for the first time was one of the most moving, emotional times I have ever had the pleasure of sharing with them. My dad is a brick. It is rare for us to see him cry. So to see the tears stream down his face made me realise what life is really all about and I haven't forgotten it since. The thought of that reminds me every day about my goal.

It was wonderful to see mum and before she had a chance to ask about our progress, I told her about my week. She is the kind of mum that feels the pain with you and will worry herself sick. I usually try to be strong when I am around her, mostly because I am scared at how I might react if I let my guard down. I don't think I will be able to pick myself up again, so for the time being, it is easier for me to act nonchalant about the subject. Take the shine off it a bit. It will be nice to have a diversion while mum is here and I thanked the universe for still being so close to her, even after six years of living interstate.

Year 2, Friday 13 October—
Daz 'n' Kaz

We are approaching 'that deadline'. November is our next appointment with Dr Fertility. January, our graduation to In Vitro Fertilisation. And with these final months comes a realisation that treatment is inevitable (as well as a sense of relief that we no longer have to have sex on demand).

October, however, is proving to be a busy month for both of us. Fez is working hard in the corporate entertainment world, selling bands and entertainment to all sorts of corporations as well as coordinating the talent to put these acts together. I am in the depths of rehearsals, and will be juggling eight shows a week up until the end of the year. This means we'll spend our first Christmas in Sydney without our families.

After the last depressing pregnancy let down, I received some good news from one of my brothers, Darren, who called to inform me that he was engaged and hoping to host a party at mum and dad's next weekend. I was surprised at the suddenness of the news and also a bit taken aback at the short notice.

Darren is the middle child (in between Steve, the eldest, and me). There's a three year, perfectly planned gap between us all. Mum didn't have to think about getting pregnant. It just happened—exactly as scheduled on the very first month of trying. Except with me it took mum two months to fall. Nothing in the scheme of things.

Darren is the kind of guy everyone likes, yet he doesn't realise it. He is simply one of the funniest, easiest and most generous blokes a person could meet, and I'm proud to say he's my brother. I still have fond memories of our childhood together. He'd take me to singing gigs when I was too young to be let into the pubs without an escort. He went straight from school to work at General Motors Holden. At the age of 16 he bought me my first second-hand car. It was a $300 orange Datsun. It was infested with spiders and broke down whenever I travelled further than 20 kilometres but I didn't care. It was my own set of wheels and the start of my teenage independence. His new fiancée, Kaz, is a lucky girl. Daz and Kaz. That will always make me laugh.

I knew it was going to be difficult for me to get the night off on Saturday, but to my amazement, I was granted leave, so I've booked myself a flight home so I can attend my brother's engagement party. It will be a whirlwind visit but means the world to my family. Fez has a function booked at which he is playing, so I am going alone.

Year 2, Thursday 20 October

Tonight's first preview of Titanic was a success. The music and score were applauded and all the right people got all the right accolades. But at the end of the day, everyone knows the ending—the ship sinks. Creating the illusion of a sinking ship on stage is practically impossible, so from that perspective, we were on the back foot as we knew the critics would have a field day with the façade of a set that simply tilted to one side, giving the impression of hitting an iceberg. Personally, I think it served better as comedy— which is awkward as it's this moment in the show when we play out our respects to those people who had actually lost their lives in the real Titanic disaster.

At least with a show like Titanic I will get to release my emotions every night when the boat sinks. I am one of the lucky ones who were lowered into the lifeboat and sings "We'll meet tomorrow" to our actor husbands left on the ship to drown. It's not really happy, uplifting stuff. I thought I'd have trouble finding the tears for eight shows a week, but tonight I just imagined singing to a child that I should have had in my twenties. I'm singing about missed opportunity and unrealised dreams and the tears just flowed.

Year 2, Saturday 21 October

Daz and Kaz's party was a wonderful affair. It was refreshingly filled with normal everyday people from Darren's work at General Motors where he met Kaz. They are a wonderful bunch and such a welcome change from the self-centred world of the arts. I enjoyed myself and was so glad I was able to go. Nothing compares to the closeness of family. In the theatre, we work so closely with our cast mates that we often refer to each other as 'family'. It's a reassuring and wonderful environment but it's nothing compared to blood. My real family will always be there for me no matter what, and they'll remember me even when my youth and talents have long subsided.

Year 2, Sunday 22 October—
Goodbye my friend

The night after the engagement party, I was invited to the house of my dear friends, Bec and Ian Blake, for dinner. They are wonderful people and, like Fez and me, they are ambitious but humble and love to travel and party. I met them at the same time I met Fez and our combined history has played a big part in our meeting. Bec and I have become particularly close since I left Adelaide and she is the only friend I ever keep in touch with regularly. I have watched her grow over the years and we've both seen each other's highs and lows. She is beautiful and intelligent while, at the same time, passionate and a little unsure of her own potential, even though to the average eye this doesn't appear evident. She keeps herself quite guarded. I can relate to that.

Each year the Blakes and Krizaks go on an annual holiday, usually somewhere in the Pacific, and laden with duty free grog. It's a special part of our lives and one that we do religiously. I remember being on holiday in January a couple of years back where I divulged our intended baby making plans to the Blakes over dinner. Of course, I always like to tell a bit more than is completely necessary and ended up informing them about my conception concerns. We weren't really 'trying' at that stage but in the back of my mind I knew we weren't being careful and had already begun to get tired of hearing people constantly ask when we were going to start a family. It was early days then and I never thought for a moment that with time, things wouldn't happen naturally. I then went on to commit the all time cardinal sin of privacy intrusion. I dismissively asked Bec if they were thinking of having children at any stage. To my knowledge, kids weren't on their menu any time in the future. At this point in the evening, Bec's gaze lowered and she got quite blunt with me.

"I really don't think that's anyone's business and it's a really personal question. I just get sick of people asking all the time."

If anyone could understand Bec's reaction, then I could. And that was the moment the penny dropped. They had been trying to conceive for six months but to no avail. I had opened up a wound. In some ways I felt comforted that I had met someone else who also had fertility concerns and who hadn't just fallen pregnant by letting 'nature take it's course' and not 'thinking about it'. That holiday, I felt closer to my friends than ever. Up until then, they hadn't told anyone they had been trying and were keeping it a secret between the two of them. Bec always said if things ever fall through for me in the entertainment industry then I should consider a career as a detective. That made me laugh. But it's true, somehow I always seem to find a way of tapping into people's darker sides.

Anyway, back to dinner. So there I was, once again sitting with the Blakes enjoying a wine and some fine food. It is always wonderful to see them and, before opening my bottle of carefully chosen Sauvignon Blanc, we decided that I should stay the night in order to get up in time to catch the first flight back to Sydney for work. Bec poured the wine and we settled in for a night of gossip and chit chat. I was feeling blissfully contented. It had been a great weekend.

"So, what's the goss?" I asked Ian as he helped himself to another glass of wine. Without a moment's hesitation, and like a scene from a slow motion blockbuster, he replied:

"Well, Bec's up the duff."

It took a moment for my brain to catch up with the words I just heard.

"Noooooooo . . . ," I said. "Really?????? . . ." I expected this to be some kind of joke and was hoping to dismiss it.

Ian and Bec looked at each other as Bec took another sip of what I now noticed was sparkling mineral water.

"Yes, it's true!" exclaimed Bec. "I'm ten and a half weeks."

I didn't know whether to laugh or cry. I wanted so much to be excited for them as they haven't been without their fair share of struggles. But at the same time, I was bitterly disappointed that I didn't have similar news to share and we wouldn't be able to go through this together. We have always joked that we would get fat together and scoff chocolate, all whilst donning a glamorous frock and stilettos.

Ian's words were still ringing in my ears. I was hoping there would be some kind of punchline but then Bec pulled out the ten week ultrasound picture and I saw their little bean for the first time.

"It's a girl," Bec said. "I just know it."

I spent the remainder of the evening in a daze, consuming copious amounts of wine with Ian, while Bec excused herself for a reasonably early night. I went to bed in their spare room with a pair of fertility dolls that Bec had been given by a friend. She placed them strategically behind my bed head in an attempt to attract the fertility gods into my life too. It had worked for them. Maybe it would work for me. I cried myself to sleep, mourning the loss of my good friend as she embarked on the journey of pregnancy and motherhood without me. In the midst of my shock over the evening's announcement, I made a pact with myself that Bec would be the person I would truly rejoice with. I know I will need to put my own struggles aside to share in her happiness. That is the right thing to do, and I am OK with that.

Year 2, 18 November—
Moving On

Mid-November and the weather in Sydney is anything but predictable. Even if it is almost warm enough to wear a dress in the evening, the wild winds have seen the end of many a festive party frock. It seems everything is out of whack, including my monthly period. Once again I am tormented with my usual 28 day period arriving a little more than two days overdue. This time I decided to take a test before my due date so I could rid myself of that niggling, rising excitement which usually ends in despair. This time was no different. To add to this I received a message on my phone that our Nov 22nd appointment with Dr. Fertility had been moved to December. More waiting.

Year 2, 25 November—
Going, going . . .

They have just announced that Titanic: The Musical will close two weeks early and the tour will be postponed due to a lack of ticket sales. The ship is officially sunk. I am secretly OK with it because it means that Fez and I can go home to Adelaide for Christmas and spend some time with our families. This wasn't the year where I wanted to be on my own, so I am sneakily relieved for the show's demise.

Year 2, Sunday 17 December—
Going, going . . . gone

Today will be the final sinking of the Titanic and aren't the media headlines having a field day with that one! It's such a shame to see a show dissolve right in front of your eyes, especially when so much time, passion and creative energy has gone into it. But hey, that's showbiz I guess, and so much goes on that is out of our hands. A show can have a good buzz around town but then fail to reach the masses of general public. It's one thing to attract hard core theatre lovers but if a show doesn't have universal appeal then it's hard to fill 1500 seats a night.

It was obvious to the cast that ticket sales had slumped; often during the matinees we were performing to as little as 10 rows of people. Sadly, this can only go on for a short period of time before the producers start to lose serious money. Subsequently, the cast were given 14 days notice and here we are at closing night already! It seems like five minutes ago that we were drinking champagne and toasting an innovative new show and relishing in our long-term employment. It just goes to show how quickly things can change. One minute you're on top of the world, the next you're back to where you started. I'd hit a lot of personal icebergs this year too. I knew the sinking feeling all too well but now it was time to say goodbye to my Titanic family and set course for a different horizon.

Year 2, Monday 18 December—
What you don't know can't hurt you

Our recent November appointment ended up being postponed due to the clinic undergoing renovations, and today was our rescheduled appointment with Dr Fertility. I can't say I took the postponement very lightly. Waiting an additional three weeks for our appointment just added insult to injury—the demise of Titanic and our appointment cancelled. Yet, once again there was absolutely nothing I could do.

Today we signed all the official IVF papers and addressed the legal issues such as the frozen embryo debate. We had to think about and agree on things like if one partner dies, and a couple has a frozen embryo in storage, does the deceased partner waive their rights for the living partner to go ahead and have his/her child? This only took a few minutes for Fez and I to discuss. If one of us was to die, we would happily want the other to give life to that embryo. We signed our signatures on the dotted line, went over our results and discussed the best option for treatment.

It was determined that we should start with a straight IVF cycle. This means that Fez's sperm motility (speed) and quantity were good, but the normal shaped sperm (which according to the assessment method used by this clinic is 15 percent) was actually down to 5 per cent. I don't know why we weren't told this in the initial testing. Was it an oversight or didn't it matter to the diagnosis and treatment? Apparently it wasn't worth mentioning.

I have a particular bone of contention when it comes to how male fertility issues are viewed. There seems to be an ego associated with men and their 'seed'. It seems OK to accept that women might have a problem and most will dismiss it as purely age related, but I was surprised at how many women were under 30 and on their second or third IVF attempt at the clinic. The problem often due to male factor infertility. Poor sperm production—motility, morphology, quantity and sometimes a lack of sperm altogether. It is more common than is widely known.

In any case, Doctor Fertility didn't see it as a setback and wants to proceed with IVF. My eggs will be placed in culture medium with Fez's sperm to allow fertilisation to take place. He wants to try this procedure before looking into ICSI (IntraCytoplasmic Sperm Injection) which is where one single sperm is manually injected into the egg to achieve fertilisation. He advised us to begin at the start line so we have somewhere to go if things fail initially. This doesn't really make great sense to me. I try to stop the negative thoughts that perhaps it is to keep us coming back for more treatment if the initial cycle fails. If we use all the bells and whistles in the first round and fail, then there's not really any point in trying again right? But who does this benefit?

I am impatient and can't see myself going through rounds and rounds of drugs when I could automatically go to the more advanced treatment. Anyway, you learn to trust in their experience and for the moment I'll run with that. It's easier to just get on with it then ask too many complicated questions at this stage. The more I ask, the more I discover and I don't want to be put off . . . I just want to get started! Ignorance is bliss. If we have to try again and again, we'll cross that bridge when it comes to it. I don't want to clutter my thoughts and start making all of this about money.

A few weeks later. I have discovered through doing some deeper research into my own test results that my FSH (Follicle Stimulating Hormone) Levels were unusually high for my age. This is something Dr Fertility also failed to point out when we got our test results back in April. FSH is responsible for producing eggs in your ovaries and the higher the hormone level, the harder the brain has to work to release those hormones. In layman's terms, it can indicate a diminished ovarian reserve. It could also mean I have a poorer response to the IVF drug treatment. My levels came back at 10.4 when I was 34. Anything below 6 is considered good, 7-9 OK, 10-13 borderline and above 14 rare success.

Of course, this is not what I would have wanted to hear and, in retrospect, it made sense that Dr Fertility had not burdened me with this vital bit of information. But if I'd known the real facts behind those numbers, would I have considered IVF at all? Was it better that I went into treatment with a positive rather than a defeatist attitude? Were these numbers reliable or could it vary from woman to woman? I don't really know why I wasn't given the hard truths. But once again, somewhere in the back of my mind, I am storing these bits of complicated information and not really processing them. It will all make sense at exactly the right time and I will know what it was I have to do. For the time being, however, Dr Fertility had just said that there was some "age related demise of the eggs".

January 11 is our first scheduled appointment with the actual IVF lab. Dr Fertility will structure all of my treatment but the actual medical processes take place in a hospital-based lab. On day 22 of my cycle, they will take my blood and wait for the results to come back. From there I will begin the suppression drugs to put my own hormones into a menopausal state in order to prepare for treatment. In the next fortnight I will immerse myself in every IVF-related book I can find and join as many an internet blog sites that I can sign up for. Oh, and did I mention no wine while preparing for treatment—Happy New Year!

CHAPTER 7

Moving on

"It won't be anytime soon, but I can see myself forming an IVF support group—one that brings people together and educates them, so that no one ever has to go through this process alone."

Year 3, Saturday 6 January— *'Tis the season to be jolly*

Christmas came and went in the blink of an eye. It was wonderful to see the family but it wasn't without its fair share of dramas. Christmas is often a time to reflect and that can be a recipe for disaster. I can't help feeling responsible for bringing out some of our family's darker traits when we come home for a visit. Quite possibly I could be overreacting to the situation, but something always seems to surface when we arrive home. We end up having to hear about everyone's indifferences. The usual problems are a result of something that has happened in someone's past. My philosophy is to dig up the dirt as quickly as possible and deal with it. Forgive, forget and get on with it. Not always a well-received approach when there is usually someone who prefers the drama rather than rational thinking. Nevertheless, as usual, as soon as we returned home to Sydney, everyone seemed to sort themselves out and things returned to normal. Go figure!

New Year was spent working. Fez had a gig with his band and I was filling in with another local party band, so we spent the majority of the night apart. Midnight rolled around and I didn't make any grand resolutions. I have already made it my motto to take things a day at a time this year. I did, however, resign myself to the fact that I never wanted to see the New Year in again having to sing 'Summer of '69'. That was painful. It's bogan retro at its best and not a song that I can relate to seeing in the new year— it's reflecting back instead of welcoming a new and fabulous year of exciting opportunity. I don't want to spend any more time looking back. Onwards and upwards, for me.

The past week has been spent lazing around and recovering from an unusually busy year. I am keen to keep work to a minimum for the first part of the year so I can focus my energies on the treatment. It won't be easy. I am a workaholic and find it hard to knock back work offers. Why is it when you start to let go of things, the offers come flooding? Typical. If, in my past, I'd been offered half the opportunities that I am being offered now, I would have dropped everything in pursuit of career recognition. Somehow the planets have miraculously aligned. How is that for timing? Just when I don't want it. Still, it's given me a new sense of confidence. Maybe this is my time. With everything else going so well around me, what's to say that our reproductive life won't also be bountiful? I'm taking this feeling and running with it. I'm on a roll and I'm not going to look back for a second while everything seems to be falling so effortlessly into place.

OK, back to the resolution. I've decided this is going to be 'the year'. I've been giving a lot of thought to how I will juggle career with motherhood. I've never really visualised myself as a stay-at-home mum forever. I don't think I would like to give up every aspect of myself. I'd like to get back on the audition circuit as soon as possible after the birth of our first child (yes, I'm still feeling incredibly optimistic). In my industry, it doesn't take long to be forgotten and although being a mum is what I want most, I think it is important to be a balanced, happy mum. I wonder if I am being selfish for wanting everything? First things first I guess.

Year 3, Monday 8 January— *Waiting for baby*

It's a matter of days until January 11—IVF orientation day at the hospital lab. I am excited but apprehensive about the long process and unsure about how I will respond to the treatment. The average cycle takes six weeks and two of those weeks are spent waiting in limbo for the blood pregnancy test.

I have become a regular visitor to various IVF blog sites and internet chat rooms where I can type all my cares away to women who are going through the process at the same time as me. Sometimes the stories are overwhelming but there seems to be a pattern emerging. Those that had success generally got there on the first attempt and were under the age of 33. For the remainder, it is not uncommon to hear of three or four failed attempts leading to a choice of either continuing with treatment, against the odds, or giving up. Most of those couples seem to choose to plough on.

There are stories of miscarriages, ectopic pregnancies (a potentially-fatal condition where the foetus implants outside of the uterus), stillbirths, loss of twins and overall higher chance of pregnancy loss in general—these intense, emotional stories keep me glued to the blog sites. For every story of triumph and joy, it seems there are at least ten heart-wrenching failures. I am morbidly addicted.

Women like these have created an institution, a virtual support network. They are there for each other from all over the world. United in their quest for a family, and struggling with the emotional impact of their infertility in a world full of pregnant bellies. It is heartbreaking.

It has just gone 1.00 am and just as I was about to pack it in for the night the title of a blog caught my eye: "How can I help my daughter. Please can someone help?" The responses are flooding in as I am sitting here, because, like me, so many other women around the world must be finding comfort browsing the internet as opposed to being left alone with their thoughts and fears. I clicked on the responses and started reading them. Before too long, the tears were welling in my eyes. An amazing woman was asking how she could reach out to her daughter in a world where nobody understands the true extent of the turmoil a woman goes through to have a child. The blog post and responses are all so moving and make me realise just how important these support sites are. I want to make a difference. It won't be anytime soon, but I can see myself forming an IVF support group—one that brings people together and educates them, so that no one ever has to go through this process alone or in a shroud of darkness. If I can make a difference, then I'll be able to find some purpose and resolution in my darkest times.

Year 3, Wednesday 10 January— *The Phantom of the ovary*

Apparently phantom pregnancies really do exist. This is when a woman is so desperate to be pregnant that she shows symptoms of actual pregnancy. Of course, I am convinced now that I've had a phantom pregnancy every month since Fez and I started trying. Even when my period arrived each time, I was sure it was implantation bleeding and proceed to squeeze my nipples to check for unusual sensitivity (which normally led to unusual sensitivity from all the tweaking!)

Multiple wasted pregnancy tests later, I knew I'd have to get help eventually. And here we are. I can't get to that IVF orientation meeting fast enough. I have resigned myself to the fact that I will never have the pleasure of spontaneously seeing those two pink lines on the stick. I'll never have that joyous realisation of being pregnant 'by accident' or celebrate with my husband over the unexpected announcement I am carrying his child. No, none of that. My immediate thought of what lies ahead of me is orientation meetings in clinical settings, where white coated doctors take my blood and pump me with hormones in an attempt to help me have a baby. Or, in one word—IVF.

Our appointment is at 10.30 am tomorrow. We will leave home an hour early to account for the flow-on of peak hour traffic. I have planned everything down to the last second. Health insurance book—check. Referral—check. Registration form—Check. Payment—'Cheque'. Emotions— Check (so far). I am ready.

CHAPTER 8

Initiation into IVF

"On the way to the car the tears continued to flow out of me. I was grieving for the wonderful chance of being able to discover the joy of pregnancy naturally—a chance I would never have."

Year 3, Thursday 11 January— *IVF Foreplay*

When we first arrived at the clinic, we were pleasantly surprised at how homely everything looked. The exterior of the clinic looked like any other house on the street and, once we were inside we were met by a young, friendly receptionist that greeted us warmly. She gathered our admission forms and we handed over the first of our $3000 instalments. It won't be until the cycle is finished that we will be able to apply for the 80% Medicare rebate required of the safety net.

We were ushered into a waiting room where we were seated with several other couples awaiting their appointments with the nurses. I couldn't help but wonder what all their circumstances were. I was momentarily distracted by a man sitting by himself, nervously holding a brown paper bag in his lap, his eyes darting all over the room without focusing anywhere in particular. I felt a small chuckle rising in my throat as I recall Fez's first experience with the small plastic container. The information in that sample bag can make or break some men and a sense of humour comes highly recommended. Looking around the waiting room, I noticed that there were no pictures of IVF babies on the walls here, just leaflets littering the waiting room tables and cabinets, offering free support and counselling sessions to couples undergoing fertility treatment at the clinic. I thought about this for a moment and was distracted again when a nurse came into the room and called out our names.

I expected our nurse to be clinical and matter of fact, but instead she was personable and thorough. She answered all my questions before the questions were even formed on my lips. She went into great detail about the side effects of the drugs and how to administer the injections. We were given all the drugs in a compact cooler bag to take home. There's the hormone suppressing nasal spray that serves to switch off my own hormones, allowing the IVF hormones to take complete control of my body. Then there's the FSH (follicle stimulating hormone) called Gonal F that is administered through injections and helps my follicles grow in my ovaries and lastly, the big shot trigger injection. This is the needle of all needles. It sends a signal to my brain to allow the ovaries to release all the carefully matured eggs and is what we'd refer to as 'ovulation' in a real monthly cycle. Except it's not just one egg that's matured, but dozens. And it's really important to avoid sex at this time or you could end up with 20 babies inside your uterus. To an infertile couple, that may sound just dandy but the reality is quite different and unfathomable.

Everything we need to know about the process was explained to us in just two hours. Fez took a keen interest in how to give me my nightly jab of hormones and we were given several practice attempts using a rubber dummy stomach and a demonstration syringe. I humoured myself when I thought of it as 'IVF foreplay'.

We left the clinic with a library of information, feeling mentally and physically prepared for the journey ahead of us. We are in this together, the day's events finalised with yet another silent tear in the car on the way home. This is it. We are now officially IVF patients.

Year 3, Friday 12 January—
Does this mean I am no longer free range?

I have to wait for the result of yesterday's blood tests to come back before I can start on the nasal spray suppression drugs. More waiting and we haven't even left the starting line yet. This is definitely no business for impatient people. Its wait until you are told. Do not proceed past GO until you get the phone call. The blood test is done to check that you have ovulated and to make sure you are not actually pregnant at the time of commencing treatment. Imagine that! Part with your $3000 and get told the next day not to bother coming back as your blood result has returned a positive pregnancy result. They say miracles happen but that would be so much more.

This fantasy manifested in my mind as I made my way to a casting audition for a television commercial. These types of castings are usually run by an agency that is hired by an advertising company to find the talent for their latest TV commercial. It's not rocket science. If you fit the physical brief, you get an audition and if they like what you do and how you look on camera they'll often call you back for a second round of auditions. For the most part, they're complete time wasters with more of a budget than they know what to do with. Being asked to come in for a 'call-back' for a non-speaking part, often just for the purpose of casting a shadow on the set is an insult to any professional. And yet, I continue to submit myself for these castings in the hope of scoring the odd job which would be financially worthwhile and grant me a bit of exposure. I try not to get too psyched up about these auditions. They were mostly a numbers game where talent is secondary.

Normally I would turn my phone off at a casting, but not today. Today I was expecting the call from the nurse informing me of my blood test results and I would be taking the call no matter what.

As I sat here with 20 other leggy blondes, my mobile vibrated and it was our nurse from the clinic calling. I caught my breath as I waited for her to tell me whether I could in fact be pregnant. Well, anything's possible right? Even though we haven't really been 'trying' this month, it only takes one time, right?

"Everything has come back fine and you're OK to commence treatment. Start your nasal spray tomorrow and remember two sprays a day, exactly 12 hours apart. I've booked you in for a follow up appointment on January 24. Good luck."

Her words were still ringing in my head. Everything had come back fine. She didn't mention whether I was pregnant or not. What about my FSH levels? Are they so high that she didn't tell me for fear it would cause undue stress? My brain was in overdrive. At that moment, my name was called and my photo taken. Moments later, I was standing in front of a camera pretending to carry a tray of drinks into a beauty spa. I had to deliver one take with a pleasant smile and one looking a "bit long in the tooth". My mind was elsewhere and as I left the room I never once wondered if I would get the job or not. I didn't care.

Year 3, Saturday 13 January—
A snort, sniff and a squeeze

I carefully unpacked my IVF 'orientation pack' and set aside the various reading materials and paperwork. Today was day one. I glanced at the schedule that our nurse had mapped out for me. Of course it is an approximate schedule, as anything could change at any time depending on how I respond to the drugs. For the time being, I am happy with a schedule. It means progress. Every day I will study it thoroughly and try to guess the due date of my baby. If I fall pregnant on the first attempt, the due date will be October 19. That seems so long away (and so long without a wine).

The morning of my first nasal spray was fairly uneventful. A few heart flutters and the gentle reminder to myself that if I am nervous about a squirt up the nose, how am I going to feel having to be injected into a roll of stomach fat every day? The spray was simply the entrée to all of this. The injections will be the main meal and, of course, the baby is my sweet reward at the end of it all. How I've always loved desserts. I decided on 11.00 am, just after I get up, and 11.00 pm, just after I finish work, for my nasal sprays which would fit in perfectly with my lifestyle and varying work requirements.

Year 3, Tuesday 16 January—
Stage 1

After a few days, the daily nasal sprays are part of the norm. I haven't been thinking too much about them. I'll deal with the side effects if they come—hot flushes, headaches and all the classic menopausal symptoms. However I hope to escape them all and sail effortlessly through my first two weeks. My house has started to slightly resemble that of a junkie—with syringes and needles stored preciously in anticipation of stage two IVF. But first things first, I have to switch off my own hormones before getting too far ahead of myself. Once I graduate to stage two I will have to go for the little blood test and then await the dreaded nurse's phone call. And to top it all off, I got the job carrying the trays. It is a TV commercial for Ocean Spray Cranberry Juice and will be filmed exactly when my proposed embryo transfer will be. So if I agree to the job, I take the chance and hope that my transfer is put back a few days. Or do I risk having to cancel the cycle for fear of being sued by the production company for breach of contract? Bitter sweet.

Year 3, Sunday 28 January—
Little red polka dots

It has been business as usual over the last two weeks with a few cover band gigs, more TV castings and the odd job as an MC thrown in. A lot of my work I manage to get through word of mouth using my own contacts. The acting auditions come through my agent. For the majority of the month I've also managed to squeeze in some rest and relaxation—quiet time, zoning out in front of the TV and giving my brain a rest. I have taken the time to gather my thoughts and work on the inner me—delving into all the stuff that makes me tick and getting to know myself better. I'm bracing myself with the emotional strength I'll need for what lies ahead.

They say that positive thinking helps with everything in life but, to be honest, it feels like anytime I've invested positive energy into anything, the opposite happens. When I dismiss something and do not let it become a part of my world and my thoughts, it more often than not works out for me. Don't ask me why. It's baffling.

Last week I was doing a gig in the city and got into a conversation with the drummer about life and personal goals. I don't know how it came about exactly but before long I was pouring my soul out to him about our desire to have a family. I think it was one of the first occasions when someone who was practically a stranger has offered me information that I could take away with me and which would have a positive effect. He said:

"Every thought has an energy. The universe will manifest those thoughts for you. Just ask for what you want and you shall receive but you must visualise yourself having already achieved that goal. You must live that life in your mind."

Those words got me thinking. Do my thoughts somehow set me up for failure? Is my image of myself as a battler—seeing the obstacles before me as negative and a challenge to be overcome—creating a pattern? This is the only way I know how to get back up and keep trying, how do you change years of conditioning?

I was inspired to try something new and different. I decided to invest in weekly sessions of acupuncture in conjunction with my IVF treatment, because I read on the internet that there is scientific evidence of greater live IVF birth rates when acupuncture is done simultaneously with a cycle. It supposedly helps with relaxation and increases blood flow to the uterus to aid in implantation of the embryo. I found an acupuncturist who operates from home, and I booked in for my first appointment.

I have been such a sceptic my whole life but where has it got me? The mind can be so powerful and as the saying goes, where there's a will, there's a way. Along with my acupuncture, I feel I needed to rid myself of any pre-determined doom. I really need to get inside of my own head and change things around a little.

During the past year many people have suggested everything from taking a holiday to turning vegan in our quest to get pregnant. They have recommended various books, movies, solutions to help me cope with our lack of prospective parenthood. They have all been well meaning, but most have been distinctly unhelpful. One suggestion came from my new guru friend the drummer who talked about the energy of thoughts. It was a movie called The Secret. With my new found positivity, I eventually found a copy of it in an obscure video shop out of town. I didn't watch it right away as I thought I needed to be in a relaxed state of mind before I would be able to benefit from the contents. I decided to watch it on the plane on my way to a corporate band gig in Singapore.

I wouldn't describe it as life changing. I will however say that it made me think long and hard about changing the way I approach my day-to-day life. Instead of expecting bad things to happen to me, I have decided to envisage only positive outcomes. Even if the outcome is not the ideal outcome for me at the time, I'll trust that it is exactly the right outcome to make way for success. It's not like fate, it's different. You have no active control over fate, but with the 'laws of attraction' that they talked about in the Secret, you apparently have the ability to control what is happening to you and to alter the outcomes. It's an interesting concept and one I believe could help (well thinking positively couldn't do harm anyway).

One of the first things I learned was how to visualise how I want to be living my life. For the best chance of success, I need to surround myself with the things that would be a living part of that outcome. Up until now I have avoided looking at baby shops to save putting myself through hell. In fact, I struggle to the extent that I can't even share in the excitement of my newly pregnant friend's shopping expeditions. It is just too painful. So now I have to challenge myself to actively become immersed in those things that I so desperately want. I have to re-discover my excitement for them by leaving my fears behind. I have decided to tackle this challenge alone.

My first visualisation experience was yesterday. As I browsed among the shops, I was attracted to a red polka dot dress. There is a simple story behind why I was attracted to the dress. Last year, one of my gorgeous girlfriends, Rockell, was two weeks away from giving birth. We were at a party for another girlfriend's baby shower and she was wearing a red polka dotted dress. I remember marvelling at her beauty and grace as she stood eight and a half months pregnant and radiant in that dress. I told myself that if there was ever a pregnant woman I aspired to look like it was her! I have held that picture in my mind for almost a year now but have always envisioned it being her in the polka dot dress, never me.

As I tentatively plucked the little polka dot dress off the rack, I automatically chose the one in a slightly larger size. Without hesitation, I took it into the change room and tried it on. I stood sideways to the mirror and pushed my hands out in the fabric to see how I would look with a bump, and I imagined myself pregnant at my girlfriend Bec's baby shower.

It was liberating. By allowing myself the simple pleasure of trying on a dress, a sense of optimism crept over me.

I bought that little red polka dot dress and hung it in my wardrobe as a reminder to me to always have hope.

Year 3, Monday 29 January—
Excuse me while I snort

My funniest recollection of this whole process to date was being onstage at a very large corporate function, and having to excuse myself at 11.00 pm to saunter off stage to snort my nasal spray. I'm sure the audience, and the band for that matter, were quite bewildered as to what it was I was so desperate to snort in the middle of our performance. Of course I never explained, I just excused myself and went about my business. Time, and hormones, wait for no-one, and this was rock and roll after all.

Since then there have been a few occasions when I have been out and the clock has struck 11. Once or twice I have been out to dinner with friends and, like Cinderella and her pumpkin, I have disappeared into the night at the sound of my mobile phone alarm. They know what I am going through but, although they listen, I don't blame them if they switch off mid-conversation when I bore them with one too many unnecessary details. It's strange to think of having a child that isn't conceived naturally. It takes the fun and excitement out of it for everyone.

Later. Since starting my IVF journey, I have been surprised at how many other women I have met that have had similar conception issues, or know someone who has undergone IVF. Yet it is still not openly talked about. You hear about celebrities who are pushing 40 talking about how they miraculously conceived twins at such a late stage in life. They just don't mention IVF, or the anguish they underwent in the process of trying to conceive. People just don't advertise it. The trouble is, when people who have been through the experience don't talk, there is nobody around to offer guidance and support to couples who are about to undergo their own fertility program. This shroud of secrecy is what has spurred me on to publish my own personal journey. Even if it reaches just a few, at least I haven't been embarrassed to admit that if all else failed, I was truly grateful for the miracle of IVF treatment.

I have just been mulling over the shroud of secrecy that surrounds IVF, when I notice the front page of the Sunday Telegraph which has a photo of Sydney newsreader Jessica Rowe holding her new baby, days after giving birth. The headline is "Jessica's miracle baby". I immediately flick open the paper to read about the arrival of her daughter Allegra. The article makes no secret of the fact that this is Jessica's fourth IVF attempt, and the joy this baby has brought to her and her husband Peter Overton, brings tears to my eyes. Somehow it just makes you that much more aware of how desperately this child was wanted when they had already been through three failed attempts. There must have been times when she would have wanted to throw it all in and give up, but she didn't and she defied the odds.

The article cites that Jessica has Polycystic Ovarian Syndrome, which causes cysts on the ovaries. I wondered if Jessica would go even further with her public admission and reach out to others in need. She certainly has broken a lot of barriers just by putting those words "IVF" in print. She has become an idol to me now and her story is another offer of hope, right up there with the polka dot dress.

Year 3, Tuesday 30 January—
Just a prick

Another blood test out of the way and I have been informed I am ready to commence the GONAL F (Follicle Stimulating Hormone) injections. I have been on the nasal spray for 12 days and it seems my hormones are 'down regulated' enough to move ahead.

I didn't get an ounce of sleep last night. It was an unusually hot, muggy night and although I am convinced I was having hot flushes as a result of the side effects of the drugs, I couldn't think about anything except the impending tummy jabs. I got up and placed a wet flannel on my forehead and eventually drifted off to sleep around 5.00 am waking to the sound of my alarm a short time later.

The blood tests are always done at 7.30 am to allow the clinic time to process the results before midday. They then phone the results through with the rest of the day's instructions. In our industry, we often don't get to bed before 1.00 am so our usual wake up time is somewhere between 9.00 am and 11.00 am. But today, the blood test means getting out of bed at 6.30 am. I made Fez drive me to the clinic. I figure if I have to go through the painful process of getting up ridiculously early every second day, then we are going to do it together.

We are all set to go and all that was left was waiting for the first injection this evening. I made sure I set my phone alarm at 7.00 pm, so we could administer the injections at the same time every evening. I still have to take the nasal spray to ensure that my own hormones remain dormant to allow for the FSH drugs to take over, so I now have three alarms set on my mobile: at 11:00 am, 7:00 pm and 11:00 pm. For me, this is the only efficient way to keep track of my drugs and remind myself to take them.

Seven o'clock rolled around and the alarm rang out a little more urgently than usual. The blood drained from my face as Fez jumped up to retrieve the injection pens from the fridge. I went and perched myself on the edge of the bath, complete with a sterile wipe and cotton wool ball to apply pressure to the injection site afterwards. This was one time in my life where I was glad to be able to grab a roll of fat from around my abdomen. This is where the jab was to take place and I made an educated guess about the more fat, the less pain. I closed my eyes as Fez finished priming the needle and I held my breath. If this was going to be painful, there would be no way I was going to look forward to another 12 days of this.

I tried to think happy thoughts but before I could even take myself off to that happy place, the procedure was over. It didn't hurt! I couldn't believe it. From what I have read, it isn't meant to be that easy . . .

"Are you sure it's gone in?" I ask Fez.

"Yes it's all in. See I can't push the button in any further."

We were both grateful that this would be a relatively easy, pain-free process. Two hurdles down and just a little under two weeks to go. Then it would be the dreaded two-week wait.

We have already decided Fez will take me away for a few days during that time, so that we can relax and distract ourselves as much as possible. I hugged Fez and we both breathed a sigh of relief. Maybe we will sail through this after all.

Year 3, Saturday 3 February—
Playing with my mind

We are four days into the jabs and onto our second injection pen. Each pen I have administers four doses of FSH, so each new pen has to be primed and then the process starts all over again. I am on 225 units of FSH, as my own levels are already reasonably high, which suggests I need a little more help to stimulate those eggs. The older a woman gets, the more FSH her brain has to produce to stimulate egg growth. Hence, because my earlier tests indicated a reading of 10.2 and some "age related demise of the eggs", I required a higher dose of artificial FSH to get my brain to start producing lots of mature eggs at once. The so-called 'normal range' is about 150 but I have met ladies on the internet blog sites who were on much higher levels, so I don't feel that abnormal.

It has been a few days since I've heard from mum. I've tried calling her a few times but she is very busy moving house with dad and getting everything in order. She promised to call me back a few times but has forgotten, and all of a sudden I feel alone. Maybe it is the hormones taking effect. I am not usually one to ask for help or support and, in all honesty, I probably don't really even need it yet. It's just that lately the smallest things will cause me to react in a way that is largely unlike me. I guess it is the hormones wreaking havoc on my body. Sometimes it is just good to know that someone is there if I need them. That someone is usually my mum. She has always been there when I've needed her and I can tell her anything. I can't take it personally when she is busy, and a reality check is just what I need to realise it isn't always about me. She has her own life too.

Last night I had a dream that we had a baby boy and named him Lyndsay. God knows why. We have never even considered that name, or any name for that matter (except for the dreaded Lyall). The dream was still vivid in my mind when I woke for my morning cup of decaffeinated tea. I had dreamt of taking my baby boy to my brother Steve's house for the first time. Steve asked me what name I had given my son and, when I said 'Lyndsay', he was horrified because in my dream that was the name he had chosen for his new son, whom unbeknown to me was not even born yet. My brother then forced me out of his home and left me standing in the driveway, alone, and with no way of getting home. I felt defenceless, excluded and alone.

What a strange dream, my brother would never do that.

Don't tell me my hormones were now intruding on my dreams? There really is no way of escaping the subconscious and today I am finding it hard to shake off the negative energy. Am I feeling somehow outcast from my own family due to not being able to produce a baby of my own? Do I feel like I am letting them down? I can't hazard a guess as to why any of these thoughts might be true but nevertheless something underlying is bothering me. Tomorrow is another day at least, and with it will come another 7.30 am blood test.

Year 3, Sunday 4 February—
Size does matter

I am getting accustomed to getting up at 6.30 am for the frequent blood tests and ultrasounds required by the clinic. I usually let Fez sleep for an additional 15 minutes, before dragging him out of bed to drive me there in peak hour Sydney traffic. I have trouble getting my head around these early appointments, let alone trying to battle for a park in the city, so Fez's duty in all of this is to be my taxi driver. He does it willingly, albeit a little bleary eyed.

Today I got to the clinic by 7.30 am and was taken to the nurse's room by 7.45 am where my blood was once again taken with another needle prick in the arm. I don't even flinch anymore. Between the blood tests, hormone injections and acupuncture I am doing, needles have become my new best friend. The acupuncture has done little to ease my anxiety levels but I will persevere for the sake of the cycle. I'll do anything to give myself the best possible chance of success. After my blood was taken, I was ushered into a smaller, darker room where I was instructed to remove my pants, sit up on the bed and cover myself with a modesty sheet. I heard a knock on the door and in walked the same nurse with a contraption in her hand that I am also well familiar with. It was the ultrasound probe. Or, as I have started referring to it as, the 'dildoprobe'.

I watched as the nurse put a condom on the probe and lathered it with a jelly-like lubricant.

"Would you like to put it in yourself?" she asked.

"No thanks," I replied. "I'll let you do the honours."

With that said, I lay back and got ready to receive the 'rod of pleasure' as I overheard another IVF patient call it a while back. There was a TV monitor above my head which showed a black and white grainy image of my uterus and ovaries.

"Ok, what we're going to do is measure the size of your follicles to see how well you are responding to the drugs," says the nurse. "We need the follicles to be at least 18 mm to harvest eggs and obviously you still have a few more days to grow yet. We'll keep monitoring you."

I continue to watch the grey mass on the screen above my head. The nurse makes little crosses next to anything that resembles a black hole. These are my follicles. The nurse begins to count.

"One, two, three, four, five on this side."

I hoped she would continue counting. The more follicles, the greater the number of eggs. She proceeded to the left ovary and I was disappointed to hear that I only had four on the left.

"This is looking fine. We will give you another scan in two days to see how they're developing. Any luck and you could be in for your egg retrieval on Monday, but be prepared it may be Wednesday. We won't know 'til your scan on Friday. At the moment all of your follicles are growing at a consistent rate and they are averaging about 12 mm."

I have read that other women have as many as 30 follicles and go on to produce at least 15 mature eggs. I was eager to get back onto the blog sites so I could compare with my internet cycling buddies. I felt a little let down. The nurse gave me no reason to question my results, but instinctively I knew that my progress was nothing remarkable. I'm a high achiever and I wanted my follicle count to exceed all expectations. What was I hoping for? A pat on the back? Some reassurance that I would soon produce a genetically sound offspring? Deal with it Deb. At this clinic I feel like I'm another patient in a long line of fertility casualties, paying my entry fees and waiting on the production line. I feel like no-one cared to invest anything more into my follicle count. It was just that—a follicle count and there would be many more to come over the next few days. I need to stop comparing my progress to everything I read on the internet. It will drive me insane.

Year 3, Friday 9 February—
Follies Bergère!

I have spent the last five days with the words "grow damn follicles, grow" resonating in my head. If the average follicle grows at 2 mm per day, then I should have been about 17 mm by today and hopefully by Monday I will have reached the desired 20 mm. I read that some women go on 'egg food' diets to enrich the quality and quantity of their eggs. Shit, last night I had ice cream for dinner and then there was that half a glass of wine at my gig the other night. I had given into temptation and was now convinced I was paying the price. I have stunted the growth of my poor eggs.

Today was yet another follicle scan. I made the earliest possible appointment as I had to shoot the Ocean Spray commercial and needed to be on set by 8.00 am. Today should technically be my final visit to the clinic before my egg retrieval operation on Monday, all being good. Fortunately, the commercial shoot would not clash with my embryo transfer after all, due to the fact that my follicles had taken that little bit longer to grow.

My blood was taken again and then it was off to the ultrasound room. The nurse made a joke as she warned me that she was about to dim the lights and create some 'mood lighting'. I also found this quite amusing.

As I lay motionless, the nurse proceeded to count the follicles on each side of my ovaries. I was amazed to hear that some had already grown to 18 mm and new follicles had emerged. Quite often it is hard to locate all the follicles as they can hide behind each other. This was comforting to know as it means there could be more eggs than first thought. The left ovary is still a little sluggish, but overall I have 12 follicles, three more than on Wednesday, with a couple that are already mature.

I left the clinic and made my way to the car where Fez was waiting to take me to my commercial shoot. The whole procedure had only taken 20 minutes and I was relieved to know I would make the shoot on time. Heaven knows I would not be needed until at least after lunch, but these people are paying you for a ten hour day and like to have you there waiting around. They feel they are getting their money's worth if they get you there from dawn I guess. I tell Fez the news that the nurse said our retrieval could be either Monday or Wednesday. I presumed I will get a call from the nurse in the afternoon to either tell me to increase my drug dosage and come back for another scan, which would delay things, or to give me a time for our day surgery on Monday. I decided to keep my phone in my jeans pocket on silent throughout the shoot. I wasn't going to miss that vibration for anything or anyone. It has been three weeks since we started this journey and I can see the light at the end of the tunnel.

The shoot itself turned out to be even more of a waste of my time than I initially thought. Basically, they hired me—the actor—so they could shoot my hand passing a glass to the two models that they have hired as Posh and Becks look-alikes. They admitted it saved time to get an actor to do this useless, degrading movement rather than hiring an extra, as we could take 'direction' better. To add insult to injury, they kept me there for the entire shoot in case they needed to use my other hand. I am ready to implode. This is a joke. I hope this negative energy won't hinder my follicle growth.

Year 3, Friday 9 February—
The year of the baby

This evening we were invited to my friend Rockell's going away gathering. All of my friends, except three, had babies last year, so the get together was at a family-friendly pub in Balmain.

I stop on the way to the pub to buy Rockell and her husband a modest bunch of flowers. They are moving to

Queensland with their eleven month old son, Mack, to buy some land and start a new life away from the rat race of Sydney. It is an exciting move for them but sad at the same time. We are a close-knit group. It had been weeks since I've been to a social occasion and I was looking forward to putting on some makeup and venturing out for a mid-afternoon meal.

When we arrived at the pub, we found our friends amidst a sea of prams and push chairs. They had taken over half the pub and their offspring were littered all over baby blankets on the floor. I carefully made my way through the gurgling babies to the equally gurgling mums and dads and found a seat away from all the commotion.

"Why did I do this to myself," I asked myself as I studied the wine list.

To have a wine, or not to have a wine? Today I NEEDED a wine. No argument with myself there. I managed to find a friend who had come alone, having recently broken up from a long-term relationship. Phew! I was safe. No chance of baby talk there.

The afternoon passed by and more families came and went. Everyone held babies and compared toilet training techniques, with photo opportunities aplenty. Fez found the boys club in the corner and managed to avoid all the fuss. It is expected that the women go all goo goo ga ga over the newborns, but this is something I couldn't bring myself to do. Just the thought of holding my friends' new offspring could wreak all sorts of hormonal havoc on me and I knew it would be best for me to avoid all emotional triggers. I have kept my emotions in check throughout our treatment, but it is confronting occasions like this that can potentially tip me over the edge and turn me into an inconsolable wreck.

Half way through my second wine, I decided to put my glass down. I didn't need alcohol to numb my pain. I had to think about my growing eggs, and think good thoughts. At that moment, Fez returned and sat down opposite me with a light beer in hand. I knew he could sense my pain and discomfort. It is a constant reminder of how we have failed at one of the most basic of human tasks—reproducing.

At the very moment I stopped feeling sorry for us, a baby was plonked on Fez's lap. I have never seen Fez hold a baby. He is always too nervous and feels clumsy, not knowing what to do. The baby was five months old and of a similar colouring to Fez with big dark eyes and thick black hair. Suddenly the tears got me. They were like a burst water main and came flooding out uncontrollably. When they started, I couldn't stop them. I wanted to run and hide but I thought that would draw more attention to my mental state, so I chose to sit here and wait for the tears to subside. How wrong I was. The sobs came next, completely involuntarily. Why didn't I run to the rest rooms straight away? My friends soon gathered around me, reassuring me that one day I would have a baby of my own. I told them that it's not like that for us and that we're going through IVF. I tried to explain that I'm on hormone treatment and that I'm hyper-sensitive at the moment. At least nobody told me to relax, or stop dwelling on it and it would happen. My friend Rockell even shared a few tears with me and made an emotional confession that she often thought about Fez and me. More sobs. The attention was making it worse. I needed to find the first available exit opportunity. It was just too much. I completely underestimated just how fragile I am.

As soon as we could, we said our goodbyes and our friends wished us heartfelt luck. On the way to the car the tears continued to flow out of me. I was grieving for the wonderful chance of being able to discover the joy of pregnancy naturally—a chance I would never have. The closest I would get is a phone call from a scientist, informing me about our little embryo's progress—whether it is dividing and what grade it is, either an A, B or C. Our little baby would have to get graded and pass so many tests just to get to the womb. I guess there is an upside, we would get a photograph of our little cells dividing. The very first images of life. Not many people get to experience that in a 'normal' pregnancy.

Back in the safe haven of our little one bedroom unit, I was beginning to get concerned that the clinic hadn't called with my test results. Each of these phone calls lets you know the next step of treatment and whether your hormone levels are in sync with the program. It said on the brochures that the nurses will always call between 2 and 3 pm. I glanced at my watch. It was 8.30 pm. Something must be wrong and they're waiting for Dr Fertility to advise them about what to do next. I was convinced. I pleaded with Fez to call the clinic for me and demand the results. Only problem was, it was almost 9 pm on Friday night, and there was no-one there. I'd been so carried away with all my problems that it had totally skipped my mind until now to call.

Year 3, Saturday 10 February—
The end of the beginning

First thing this morning, I got Fez to pick up the phone and dial the clinic. He went through the identification process and eventually a nurse came back to him with yesterday's results. As it turns out, they were trying to contact me but my mobile phone was saying it was out of range. Fez furiously scribbled down a series of dates and times on a piece of paper as I listened intently, bursting with curiosity. Fez put the phone down and informed me that all was going to schedule and we were to make our way to the day surgery on Monday at 8.00 am as planned.

Tonight was my final night of the FSH injections, and the final trigger injection should be administered at exactly 8.30 pm tonight. I am told to fast from 12 midnight Sunday night and to bring the semen sample to the hospital when we come. My stomach flipped. In exactly 48 hours I will be having my first anaesthetic and a needle will pass through my vaginal wall and into my ovaries to suck out my eggs. Hopefully, the needle will miss all my other internal organs and I will awake without any major pain, with a number of at least 10 scribbled on the back of my hand. This will be my first indication into how well my ovaries have performed, as well as the number of eggs collected.

My brain processes every possible disaster scenario. And then I am once again overcome by emotion. I have sailed through three weeks of treatment and all the hurdles that I envisioned happening, have not evolved. I feel incredibly lucky but the journey is yet to begin. I called my mum and sobbed into the phone. She was sobbing too, expecting me to give her the bad news that the cycle had been cancelled. I controlled my own tears long enough to tell mum the good news, and we cried again together. This is going to be the most important two weeks of my life.

Year 3, Sunday 11 February—
Shattered glass

Today was officially the final day of drugs, and what a day it was. I feel blessed that I have survived this far. The trigger injection was this evening, and I knew that when that was over, we would be left with the emotional aftermath of the two week wait. To fill in the time, we have arranged to go away up the coast for two days and I have scheduled in a job shooting another TV commercial. That will help to keep my mind occupied and distracted. I can't imagine the sheer horror of my period arriving in that two weeks and the realisation that all the work up until now was in vain.

Injection time (8.30 pm) rolled around and Fez dashed back from a gig in the city to administer it. We had 20 minutes to mix the powder with the solvent solution, give the injection, and get Fez back to work. We were on a tight schedule but I didn't trust myself to do it alone.

The trigger injection comes in three glass vials that need to be broken before drawing up the fluid and mixing it with the powder. It's quite complex in comparison to the diabetic style pen we are accustomed to. Fez broke the top off the first vial and, to our horror and disbelief, the glass top shattered, leaving Fez with two nasty gashes in his thumb. My heart stopped beating. I took the remainder of the vial from Fez and checked to see if the contents were still intact. On closer observation, I noticed some shards of glass amongst the powder. This was not good. I bandaged Fez's thumb, and we continued to break the vials and draw up the injection solution. I tried calling the clinic to find out what I should do about the broken glass, but being a Saturday night, the clinic was unattended. We would have to decide if we were going to proceed with the possibility that tiny pieces of glass could have penetrated the solution.

I felt my heart race as the implications of injecting a drug contaminated with fine splinters of glass, entered my mind.

"Should I be doing this? Why wasn't there a damn emergency number to contact? Hell knows."

I was getting agitated. We attached the needle to the solution and, on careful inspection, decided to proceed with the trigger shot.

Fez reassured me that the eye of the needle is so fine that it would not allow any glass to be injected into my blood stream. I took a deep breath and had the shot at 8.40 pm, ten minutes late. It wasn't a joyous end to the drugs. I felt anxious and scared.

Hours have passed now. I am still breathing and my heart rate is normal. I will be ovulating in 36 hours. Before I got into to bed, however, I leaned over my bedside table to put my tea cup down and found an old Christmas card wedged between the wall and the cabinet. It was a card Fez had given me a few years back. It said:

"Looking forward to spending next Christmas with our little one."

It's the first time he had ever acknowledged us actually having a family. At times during this past year I wondered if he really wanted it as much as me, but now I am sure. Men suffer silently. They don't always talk about how they feel as a partner in all of this. They are there to prop us up and lend a sympathetic shoulder when we encounter the invasive procedures and emotional setbacks. I wondered if Fez ever cried alone at night. I guess I will never know.

Year 3, Monday February 12 February 8am— *D Day*

Today was the day of Egg Retrieval, or Oocyte Retrieval as the scientists call it. We arrived at the day surgery at 7.30 am and took our place in the waiting room, which was unusually quiet. We must have been the first patients for the day. The receptionist looked up at us over her glasses and instructed Fez to deliver his sample through the lab doors. With IVF, you are constantly asked to confirm your name and to deliver specimens directly to the scientists yourself. This eliminates any possibility for error. It is a very delicate process. After filling out legal submission forms, I was given a hospital wrist band and told to take a seat in the deathly cold waiting room. There was a stale smell resonating throughout the room which was making my stomach churn.

I was ushered into a tiny cubicle, instructed to remove all my clothing and jewellery, and put on a hospital gown. I was given a hair net, booties and a plastic bag to place my belongings in. Suddenly I felt as if I was going to my death. My mind played out my worst fears in my head—I don't wake up from the anaesthetic and Fez is slumped over my clinically dressed body, having being handed a plastic garbage bag with the last items of clothes in it, that adorned my body only moments before. Kind of like a soldier of war but without the state funeral.

I shook my head and diverted my attention back to my eggs. I was assured the operation only took ten minutes and in a way I was glad that I didn't have to go through the humiliation of being conscious while they lifted my legs up into stirrups and gave me the antiseptic vaginal wash. Hell, it's worth being under just to avoid that. The anaesthetist introduced himself and after I was weighed, he told me the cost for his services and probed me about my health insurance. With my health insurance rebate, I would only be a little out of pocket for his services which seemed like chicken feed in comparison to the thousands we'd already handed over for one chance at IVF. I was again asked to repeat my name and to confirm the procedure I was about to have. Far too many questions. Not even minutes passed and Dr Fertility came into the room to collect me and ask me how I was feeling. He was equally clad in full hospital attire, but with a surgical mask. I was relieved to see his familiar face. Up until now I'd never noticed his tanned skin and comb-over hair style. His eyes were sparkling and he looked fresh and positive. I was wheeled into the operating theatre and was surprised to see half a dozen doctors, nurses and scientists. Perhaps this procedure ran more risks than I had given it credit for. I suddenly remember last night's dream:

There was a production line of infertile women who were banked up in a hospital corridor awaiting their egg retrieval. There wasn't nearly enough room, so I, being second in line, had to wait in the operating theatre doorway, and watch as the woman before me had her eggs extracted. Suddenly, I heard a flatline, and the woman's heart stopped. No attempts were made to resuscitate her and no urgency was displayed by the hospital staff. I heard the words: "Don't worry, you can't win them all", as a sheet was placed over the woman's head and she was declared dead. The attention then turned to me and the scientist called "Next!". After witnessing this horror, I desperately tried to release myself from the bed but was somehow strapped down and unable to move.

I eventually woke from that dream, with my heart racing and in a cold sweat. Perhaps I was a little more anxious than I first thought. Too late to back out now.

I was given a mild sedative to relax me before the anaesthetic was administered. The anaesthetist was careful to explain everything I could possibly feel as the drug filled my veins. He said the worst part would be the injection going into the vein, which didn't faze me at all. After all needles are now my best friends.

The next thing I remember is waking up in the recovery room with someone shouting my name over and over again. I woke reluctantly. It was the best nap I had had in ages. The nurse asked me my name—once again—and I muttered, "Sandra Dee". She looked at me bewildered. Of course I was only joking. I was just high on life, having come out of the anaesthetic in one piece. Unfortunately, having a quick wit isn't always well received and I was kept in the recovery room a little while longer than the average patient—so they could determine whether I was still under the effect of the anaesthetic or just plain loopy. What the nurse didn't realise was that I was euphoric from not only having woken up, but also from seeing the number 15 scribbled on my left hand. I had produced 15 eggs. Those damn follicles had grown after all.

Year 3, Tuesday 13 February—
Eggs Eleven

This morning I woke at 7.00 am. Even though I could allow myself a sleep in this morning, it's no use, I couldn't sleep. The lab would be calling at 10.00 am to give us the update on our eggs. We were told that as this was our first IVF cycle there may be a chance that none of those 15 eggs would fertilise at all. Once again, it is another waiting game.

At ten minutes to 10.00 am, my mobile phone rang. I didn't recognise the caller ID. I answered the phone and it was the scientist from the lab.

"We have good news. Eleven of your eggs have fertilised and we're on track for your embryo transfer tomorrow. Dr Fertility would like you to be here by 7.30 am tomorrow morning. Make sure not to wear any perfumes or deodorants as it can interfere with embryo development."

The scientist spoke softly and was very matter of fact. I strained to hear every word and didn't want to miss any important information.

"Does that mean we have done well? Is this good?"

"Yes, that's an excellent result," she said.

I put the phone down and jumped up and down with excitement. "We've got 11 fertilised," I screamed to Fez.

Fez looked genuinely amazed. I hugged him and a solitary tear trickled down my right cheek. I thought to myself, I must ring Mum and tell her the good news, and while I'm there I'll text my girlfriends too. For a moment I forgot about the stinging pain in my abdomen from yesterday's operation, and I spent the rest of the afternoon on the internet, informing my blog friends around the world of our good news.

Year 3, Wednesday 14 February—
And then there were two

Ironically it was Valentine's Day today, as well as the morning of our embryo transfer. The alarm woke me at 6.00 am and I had trouble getting Fez to respond to the early wake up call. I let him lay in bed while I showered and got dressed. Fifteen minutes later, Fez dragged himself out of bed in a sleepy daze, and we left our apartment at exactly 6.40 am.

I was much more relaxed about today's procedure. I had been told it was very quick and involved placing the embryo into my uterus through a fine catheter inserted via the vagina. Apparently it causes no more discomfort than your average pap smear. I hoped that we might get to see our little embryo under the microscope.

Moments after leaving our apartment, Fez's face drained of all colour and he screamed out a profanity. He had forgotten to pick up his keys on the way out of the door, and subsequently left us locked out with no way of getting back in again. Not only that, but we didn't have the car keys either so we were stuck for transport with 40 minutes to get to the lab in peak hour traffic. Fez's face was white, mine went bright red. I was so God damn angry. Why the hell did he forget to pick up the keys? Doesn't he know how important this appointment is? This couldn't be happening. I was so angry with him I couldn't even respond.

"We'll have to get a cab," I proclaimed in a sharp tone.

A cab would cost us $130 for a round trip and a locksmith another $80. All the money I had saved on insurance had just been wasted in that one careless second.

Luckily a taxi arrived within minutes, which is no surprise really. It's funny how taxis always turn up on time when there is a substantial fare in it for them. Our taxi driver's name was Sunny and he was incredibly chirpy for someone who had started work at the crack of dawn. We arrived at the day surgery with five minutes to spare and Sunny offered to wait around for us and give us a lift back home.

The waiting room was full to the brim and I recognised another couple who were in for their egg retrieval on the same day as me. The lady recognises us too and approaches us to ask how many eggs we collected. I welcomed the chat, even though to someone else this could be interpreted as intrusive. I explained that we got 15 eggs and that 11 had fertilised. I was keen to know what their result was. Actually, I was just keen to talk to someone! They only got three eggs and this was their third IVF attempt. They were eager to exchange information which made a welcome change from the evasive stares from the other women I had met at the clinic. Nobody spoke there. It was as if everyone was too ashamed. It really affected me how these women couldn't unite in their fears and turn to one another for support.

At exactly 7.30 am we are taken into a smaller room where the lab scientist explained the progress of our embryos. Two have divided into 4 cells, which is normal for a 48 hour period, but the others are looking a bit slow to multiply. Two of the 'slow' embryos showed potential and they would be kept for another day to see if they continued dividing. Potentially we had four embryos at the day two stage of development. One earmarked for transfer today, one frozen, and two kept under close observation. Out of those 11 we had yesterday, only two have progressed today. The rest would be donated to science at our request.

The transfer room was tiny and my first thoughts are that we couldn't possibly be doing the transfer in this tiny, restricted space. I then saw the same 'dentist's' chair and the embryologist asked Fez to take a seat next to this chair. The room was roughly the size of our bathroom. Not exactly the kind of environment I wanted to be impregnated in. Where was the soft music, the burning incense? Oh yes, that's right, strong odours interfere with embryo quality. I settled into the cold, steel chair and Dr Fertility came in to tell me once again to remove my clothing from the waist down. This was the first time Fez had witnessed exactly how intrusive this process has been for me.

Fez placed a firm hand of support on my upper arm. My legs went into the stirrups, I placed the hospital sheet discretely over my private parts and waited for Dr Fertility to return. There were now four of us in the tiny insemination room, and the embryologist asked for confirmation of my name once again. She then asked me to look at the screen above our heads, and next to my scribbled surname was our little four-cell embryo. Four perfect circles, overlapping each other. We were amazed. It looked exactly like the photos in the books but the hopes riding on this one are so much more. The embryo was placed into the tiny catheter and deposited straight into my uterus, a procedure not dissimilar to a pap smear. Within seconds it was all over.

"That's a very good looking embryo," Dr Fertility commented, and I smiled.

"So, it looks normal?" I asked, searching for some kind of affirmation that it has a good shot of making it.

"Yes, very good indeed", he replied with a genuine fascination.

This man really loves his job, and it was never more evident to me than at that moment. Even as he sat staring at the entrance of my womanhood, he was basking in the glory of his job—creating life. Dr Fertility is like a surrogate father to our potential child. Sometimes it takes more than two to make a baby.

I pulled on my jeans and was reassured that the embryo couldn't fall out. Dr Fertility advised me to carry on living as normal, which includes having sex as it can even promote the embryo to implant. Before implantation can happen though, our little four-cell embryo will have to divide to another 16 cells, break out of its outer shell and snuggle into my uterine lining. In the meantime, I need to insert progesterone pessaries, morning and night for the next two weeks. These look like giant tampons with an applicator and are filled with the hormone progesterone. They will keep my womb lining rich and full of blood, ready to assist the all-important implantation. Without the optimum environment, no matter how good an embryo is, it won't survive if it can't latch on and form the early stages of the placenta.

During the long taxi ride home, I called mum and breathed a sigh of relief that it was all over. I have triumphed. Sunny, our taxi driver, took great pride in telling us all about the nudist beaches of Sydney, and as my mind drifted off amidst the buzz of morning peak hour traffic, I subconsciously rubbed my tummy, realising this is the closest I have ever been to being pregnant. I lit a candle of hope in my heart.

Year 3, Thursday 15 February—
The two week wait

It's a brand new day, and with it came a new strain of anxiety brewing inside of me. I awoke to the wonderful thought that there were no more injections, no more nasal sprays and no more early morning blood tests with the occasional dildoprobe thrown in. It didn't stop me from waking up at 7.00 am again though. The first thing I noticed was a nagging feeling in my stomach and it took me a moment to realise what was bothering me. I have read about this condition all over the internet blog sites. It's referred to as the dreaded 'two week wait'. It's the period of time in your treatment where there are no daily updates of your progress, no phone calls from the lab and no guarantees that all the hard work has paid off. It was now in the hands of the gods.

I decide to get out of bed and log onto my internet support group. There were countless stories of women struggling with the agonizing two week wait, deliberating over whether to do a home pregnancy test before their scheduled blood pregnancy test was due. Mine is scheduled for two weeks after embryo transfer, on Wednesday the 28 February. What on earth am I going to do to keep myself occupied for the next 14 days?

It will feel like an eternity. There's not much in the business diary to keep me occupied either. Fez and I have grown accustomed to the beginning of the year 'slump' in work bookings. We plan for it in advance every year. We'd have a boomer November/December, make two thirds of our yearly income in that period and then put any surplus cash away for the new year. We think of it as our 'annual leave' where we get paid for taking a bit of a break. Planning ahead financially is imperative.

Technically, my period is due on the Monday 26 February, before my official test, which the clinic does on purpose to ensure you don't test too early and get your hopes up. Most women experience their period before getting to their blood test but are still made to go in for the blood results as a routine part of the process. That would be agony of the highest order.

There is no point looking for early pregnancy signs yet, it will be at least seven days before I can possibly feel anything. That won't stop me researching what I can possibly feel in a week's time however. Implantation cramps, sore nipples, even possible nausea. All of them, the same side effects I could experience from the progesterone pessaries. Damn this stuff knows how to play with my head. There is no way of detecting if I am pregnant until around 24 February or unless, God forbid, my period does arrive on the Monday before my 'bloods' are taken. Pregnant until proven otherwise. That is my new motto. I might as well settle in for the long haul. This is why everyone calls it the agonizing wait. This is by far the hardest part of the journey to date.

I ventured downstairs to check my neglected mailbox. I figured this should keep me distracted for at least half an hour while I sorted through all the unpaid bills and reminder notices. Amongst the mountains of envelopes, there was a letter from my local doctor's surgery. I opened it to read that it was one of those friendly but persistent reminder letters to attend the surgery for my annual pap smear. I went upstairs and placed the letter on my fridge as a reminder to myself to schedule an appointment. I have finally conquered my fear of the pap smear and seeing as this is the month of the legs in the stirrups, why torture myself about it now? I had a private giggle at the thought of the old me. The girl who would nearly faint at the thought of having to pick up the phone and make that appointment.

Year 3, Friday 16 February—
Blast(ocyst) from the past

It turns out that one of the two slow dividing embryos we had in the lab decided to get a move on and made it to a four-cell embryo overnight. The embryologist called this morning and left a message on my voicemail. I am delighted to know we have another little embie for cryostorage or, as we refer to it, 'putting it in the freezer'. We now have two embryos in storage, ready for a Frozen Embryo Transfer (FET) if we need to progress to a second cycle.

Over the past month I haven't really felt like doing too much. Most social occasions can be avoided with some lame excuse, but once in a while an event comes up that we both decide we should make an appearance at.

Earlier this evening I got a phone call from an old work colleague informing me that she was friends with an old friend of mine that I hadn't seen in ten years. She suggested we all meet up over a drink. It felt odd that after all this time we were being given an opportunity to see each other again. It had been a rough end to the relationship all those years ago. We were childhood best friends and grew up in each other's pockets. We shared the kind of things that stay with you for life. I always thought of her on her birthday and daydreamed about the moment we would meet again, and now here it was.

We agreed on a meeting place where we could all go for a casual drink. I must admit I am nervous. I am aware that my long lost friend has been having her own fair share of fertility problems through information our mutual friend had provided, but I am not sure of how open she will be to share those struggles. I have just realised the meaning behind this meeting. Our mutual friend has carefully planned this reunion. She is hoping that our infertility may open the door to rekindling the friendship and finding some common ground again after all these wasted years. Of all the things that could bring us back together, I never thought in a million years, that it would be our yearning desire to have a baby.

Year 3, Tuesday 20 February—
Does time heal all wounds?

I was nervous about the meeting. What should I wear? How should I greet her? Keeping in mind the awful words I spat at her in an Adelaide pub almost ten years ago, would she still be angry? As Fez and I drove into the city I decided I would play it cool and wait for her to initiate the conversation.

I was waiting like an eager spectator as my old friend and new friend greeted each other enthusiastically. Any moment now, they would acknowledge me and invite me in. I waited. I waited some more. I felt myself go red. My mind was racing. I considered bailing out and making a swift exit. At that moment, our mutual friend turned and said:

"You remember Deb don't you?"

"Oh of course," she said, as if up to that moment she had been completely oblivious to me being there.

I came to the realisation that the waiting was a show of power over me to let me know that she was in control of the situation. I surrendered and we attempted to engage in a fake embrace. Things were still icy after all this time. It's amazing how childhood competitiveness can impact on an adult's life. Those memories of inadequacy can stay with you forever.

We sat down and ordered a round of drinks. Both friends made excited chatter and I tried to think of ways to force myself into the conversation. Then it dawned on me, my old friend was also drinking water. Everyone else had ordered wine. My mind took a moment to catch up to the reality. Lately, it seems that I am like a lucky charm for every other couple trying to get pregnant. I almost can't go out anymore for fear of being stuck in a social occasion where a friend makes the wonderful announcement that she is expecting. It was about to happen to me again now. I just knew it. This was why she agreed to meet up again—to leave me sitting there with egg on my face—to win the race before me—to bask in her glory. And there was nowhere I could run and hide.

As I made idle chatter with my old friend's husband, I strained to hear what was being said in hushed voices between my two friends. I heard the word "little bean" and before I could delve any further, they were embracing and I heard the word "congratulations". I knew exactly what was evolving in front of my eyes. My old friend was of course four weeks pregnant on her very first IVF cycle . . . and she got 18 eggs. My old friend had come here to share the news with our mutual friend, but somewhere deep inside me, there was a niggling knowledge that this announcement had also been for me. Another friend has jumped on the baby train and I am left standing waiting for the bus. Story of my life. After the excitement of the announcement died down, my old friend excused herself and said she had to get to another social engagement. We barely spoke a word to one another. Her mission was accomplished and, as I walked back to my car, I felt like the competitive loser.

Year 3, Wednesday 21 February—
Seven days and counting . . .

After just one week, the two week wait has evolved into everything I dreaded it would be. Hours are beginning to feel like days, and days feel like weeks. Sometimes it is hard not to watch the clock tick. Never have I wanted time to pass so quickly. Up until now, I had things to do, appointments to keep, and daily tasks to keep myself occupied. Now I am left with just 'what ifs'. I praise each passing day for being closer to the moment of truth.

Subconsciously, I have already planned my pregnancy demise. It involves an incredibly expensive bottle of wine and a healthy hangover the following morning. How I long for a glass of wine to take the edge off the situation. Fez has done his bit in the cycle. He has produced a healthy specimen and he is now free to resume life on the dark side—by that I mean, dark spirits and anything else toxic that he can lay his hands on in liquid form. I am slightly envious of his new founded freedom. Me, on the other hand, I have to refrain from alcohol altogether, avoid hot tubs and spas, eliminate caffeine and stop exercising to give myself the best possible chance for our little embryo to implant. Anything less than that and I would blame myself for getting a negative result. It definitely isn't easy. It is a constant reminder of the process and everything that I have had to go through for the dangling promise of a potential pregnancy.

Aside from being completely pregnancy obsessed, Fez and I are holding up OK. I still feel pretty alone throughout this whole waiting period. I can put on a fairly good poker face but I'm lying if I don't admit that every waking moment is spent wondering if this is going to be it or not. It's like being in a pressure cooker waiting for the steam to erupt. I think Fez is preparing himself for the aftermath. If he is, he's not talking about it either. We're just going about our business trying to remain as normal as possible. Easier that way. Don't have to talk about the 'what ifs'. They can just fester in my subconscious. We haven't had sex since the transfer, in fact we haven't had a lot of sex since we stopped trying to fall pregnant naturally. I could analyse this part of our relationship over and over and look for all the trouble spots but the truth is, I think we're doing just fine under all the strain and circumstances. We are intimate with each other in so many ways. I just don't need the added pressure of feeling sexy at the moment. I don't feel sexy. My own hormones have been switched off for a while now. I want to just exist at this level of numbness for the time being. It's safer.

Year 3, Thursday 22 February—
Escape . . . ?

It was the week for baby announcements. A friend called and refused to leave messages on my voicemail. Eventually I answered the phone to what appeared to be another "we wanted to tell you in person" that they are pregnant. Oh joy. Another emotional scar. Then there's the friend who, at 41, went on her honeymoon and fell without trying. The list is endless. It wreaks havoc with your emotions. So easy for everyone else, so damn hard for us. This two week wait is definitely getting to me. I'm not feeling very optimistic.

Fez and I planned to go away for a few days to get some relief from the fertile outside world. We booked a little Bed and Breakfast, just 45 minutes from Sydney to give ourselves some time to do nothing and enjoy each other's company. The weather had been beautiful and our accommodation was beachfront so we were much looking forward to it.

I am still only 8 days past transfer. Just over half the waiting is over. We arrived at our beachfront B&B to find we had been blessed with torrential rain and with no choice other than to lock ourselves inside until the weather passed. This left me of course with far too much time to contemplate the 'what ifs'. Should I be experiencing implantation cramps by now? Should my boobs be sore? They were definitely bigger. However, unfortunately the progesterone pessaries I was inserting morning and night also replicate symptoms of pregnancy. There is never any way to know how you are doing and I've spent countless nights surfing the blog sites for some indication that no symptoms could also be a good sign.

Our B&B hosts were friendly, if not a little too friendly at times, and we were given some local information on what we could do if the weather fined up. There was a spa out on the lawn area which would have sufficed in the terrible weather, but spas are of course off limits to pregnant women. So is the chilled bottle of champagne that is sitting in the fridge tempting me. I asked Fez to enquire whether we would be able to alter the spa's thermostat so we could have a cool spa at least. Always putting my little growing embryo first. Oh how I wish I had a camera inside me showing me all the little developments, day by day. Has my embryo died already or is it burrowing into my nice thick progesterone-coated lining? My attention came back to the spa. As the conversation with the B&B hosts continued, it was clear they are not going to answer Fez's question without a reason as to why we would like to turn the heat off. Fez stumbled on his words and looked at me. We were lost for an explanation. Oh, what the hell.

"I may be pregnant," I blurted out, thinking that this would put a stop to the inquisition.

"Oh, well you shouldn't use the spa at all then," our host said defiantly. "Why don't you pop over to the chemist and get yourself a pregnancy test, and then you'll know for sure," she continued with heightened enthusiasm.

"Thanks for the suggestion," I said as I managed a wry smile. I have been trying to avoid those damned pee-on-a-stick home pregnancy tests for a week, and now I was being coaxed into buying one for the sake of a leisurely soak in the spa on a winter's day. Those damned tests have never been kind to me. Why would that change now? Taking one this weekend would only destroy my dream and the glimmer of hope that not knowing for another week will bring.

Eventually I had to tell the pestering host that I am an IVF patient and things don't quite work the same as a natural pregnancy, otherwise her questions wouldn't have let up. She was making all kinds of suggestions about how we could go to the lovely country stalls and buy ourselves some baby clothes. I virtually yelled at her: "I AM NOT YET PREGNANT". But this didn't seem to be getting through. She then proceeds to drag me indoors and show me her 11 month old twin granddaughters, conceived naturally of course. The thought entered my mind to pack up and get the hell out of there. They wouldn't need to know. We'd just put it down to the bad weather. People just have no idea, even when you spell it out to them.

After what seemed like an intrusive hour of questioning, Fez and I decided to lock ourselves safely in our room for the night and enjoy the serenity. It was hard to keep my mind occupied with the silence so deafening and the words of our 'friendly' hosts ringing over and over in my head. Where exactly was that chemist? Could I walk there now? Would it be open late at night? I decided to fill the lurching obsession in my stomach with food. I seem to be doing that a lot lately. I dislike the way I look in the mirror after having gained five kilos from the fertility drugs, but I reassure myself it will soon disappear and I grabbed another chocolate biscuit from the fridge—and then another. The packet is now empty and I am even more depressed. Depressed from having no control over my body. Depressed over food, over this uphill battle to be able to have a baby, over Fez not being able to have a child of his own, over watching him try to stay strong for me.

Year 3, Friday 23 February—
First response

I awoke this morning and made a mental plan for the day. Perhaps a trip to that chemist for some Vaseline. Overnight I have acquired a swollen clitoris. It felt as if it had been trying to grow overnight. It is of course a side effect of the drugs. Perhaps I am turning into a man. I can hardly walk, so a trip to the chemist was confirmed as the first stop of the day.

Fez waited outside for me as I surveyed the shelves for Vaseline. I had already stalked out the home pregnancy kits. There was one for $13 that was called 'First Response', and could detect hCG in your urine up to seven days before a missed period. hCG stands for 'Human Chorionic Gonadotrophin' which is a hormone that is released by the placenta into a woman's bloodstream and subsequent urine once an embryo has implanted. Perfect. I bought it discreetly with the aim of deciding what to do with it later. It would take the place of those chocolate biscuits. Far less calories. I did the sums in my head and worked out that I was technically only three days away from an impending period. I could do the test tomorrow morning and be put out of my misery.

The rain continued to pelt down and our plans of exploring the local area on foot turned into another nightmare encounter with our B&B hosts offering unprompted advice and more questions. We decided we would be safest back in our room and that's where we stayed. Fez was anxious to check his emails and I was having withdrawal symptoms from not being able to get my daily fix of positive mental attitude from my internet blog friends. I was desperate and anxious and bored. This treatment has preoccupied my life for the past three months and I find no relief in any other part of my life. Every morsel of hope is aimed towards having this baby.

As night approached Fez decided to take a walk and get some dinner for us both. We decided on pizza from the local café. I stayed in. Sometimes the thought of putting on a bra to go out is overwhelming. My boobs are so heavy and big that I just can't hide them no matter what I do and I am far more comfortable hanging around the house braless, and in an old baggy T-shirt. Left alone with my thoughts, I found myself contemplating the home pregnancy test. I had a window of opportunity to do it, while Fez was out. I knew he didn't want me to do a test, so if I was to do it, I would have to do so on the quiet. I spent a few moments going through the 'what ifs' in my head.

What if it was negative? Would I crumble into despair for the next week before my blood test? Would I be able to cope? I took a deep breath and decided that I would do the test and, if it was negative, I would not lose hope. It could simply mean it is just too early to test.

I reached into my bag and took out the instructions on the test, as if on autopilot. It said first morning urine is preferred for early testing but that it can in fact be done at any time of the day. I took the test out of its foil packaging and locked myself in the bathroom. I peed on the stick for exactly five seconds and placed it on the flat bathroom vanity unit. It was different from some of the other tests I have taken, but the result is the same. It says to wait no less than three minutes and no more than ten minutes, to get an accurate reading. I watched as the pink dye washed over the test and a line appeared almost immediately in the control test window. This meant the test was operating correctly. I waited 30 seconds with my eyes squeezed shut. I don't think I was breathing. My hands started to shake. For a brief moment I prayed for a miracle. Suddenly there was a knock on the door and Fez had returned with the pizza. I shouted out to him that I was having bowel problems and that I'd be out in a second. He didn't respond. I diverted my eyes back to the test. The window is white. There's nothing there. I stared at it blankly. I stared at it in disbelief. All the weeks of injections, drugs, scans, operations, blood tests, the money spent, hopeful calls to mum . . . all come down to this moment. And there it was. Nothing. Not even a faint line. I hung my head and placed it between my knees, all the while I was still sitting on the toilet. The test claimed to be 99% accurate. Now all I was left with was 1% of hope.

Strangely, I didn't shed a tear. I am used to these tests coming up negative. I guess I was in shock for the most part of the next 30 minutes. I tucked the test inside my jacket pocket and made my way out of the bathroom to find Fez sitting outside on the grass, dividing up the slices of pizza.

"Hurry up," he said. "Yours is getting cold!"

I took my seat on the grass, next to my glorious husband. Fez has never asked for much in life. He makes decent money and still manages to have a decent amount of down time. He'll do anything for anyone and would give away his last penny if he could. Well, that was of course until he met me. I took a slice of greasy pizza and put it up to my lips, trying to play happy families. I made conversation with Fez, but I don't remember what we talked about. I wondered if I should tell him what I'd done.

After dinner, we went for a walk on the beach. The reality was beginning to sink in and I was damn mad at myself for destroying our embryo's hope prematurely. I could have sworn I felt little cramps in my side this morning. I was almost certain it was implantation cramping. Maybe it was the embryo switching off the light. They say sometimes your egg just doesn't have enough battery power to sustain its own cell growth. I thought ours was a good one. Dr Fertility had said it was a "fine looking embryo". What the hell had happened?

We stopped momentarily on the beach and Fez put his arms around me. Here we go. I felt the tears well up from a place so deep in my soul that I knew this kind of pain would take a long time to subside. Maybe months. I couldn't look him in the eye but I couldn't live with this secret either. I told him. For a moment he was in disbelief. Like me, it took him a while to process the implication of what I had just told him.

"Are you sure," he asks.

I pulled the test out and explained that it was an early detection test and 99% accurate. I couldn't bear to just throw the stick away. Fez paused for a moment and in his usual matter of fact way, he said:

"Oh well, we'll just have to try again my darling."

I cried when all I really wanted to do was scream. I wanted to howl. Fez braced himself to once again be my rock. I could tell he was bitterly disappointed. He watched me go through this. He was so careful with those injections and watched me wince every time my alarm went off to signify it was time for another jab. He held my hand when I thought I was going to die when they put me under anaesthetic. He gave me confidence when I thought we would not get many eggs, and he rejoiced with me when 11 of the little buggers fertilised. It is the end of the road as we know it this time. We packed up our things and left the holiday house. There was no reason to be there anymore. Being left alone with just my thoughts was too painful. At least at home we would have distractions, and I would be able to find some solace on the internet. We left without telling the B&B hosts and we drove through the dark, quiet night.

Saturday 24 February—
Pee stick addict

Being alone with just your thoughts is a confronting, lonely experience. I have read extensively on the beneficial effects of positive thinking. I'm at the stage now where I need a manual on how to attain that positivity in the constant face of adversity. I can't find a positive anywhere in all this madness. Did I really believe it would work the first time? It worked for my friend. But she went to another clinic which is more expensive and supports day five blastocyst transfers. I liken it to winning the lottery. IVF is a numbers game. The odds suggest that IVF patients who are destined to have success do so within four full treatment cycles. But I feel that the more attempts, the more likely we are to hit the jackpot. I am not about to give up, but instead of getting easier, this will only get harder. I am becoming more obsessive, hanging onto the faint hope that perhaps the urine test was wrong.

I logged onto my fertility blog site and posted my latest events on the web. Within minutes I had a flood of replies from my cycle buddies around the world. They kept reassuring me that the tests could be wrong and I am more likely to get a false negative than a false positive. I felt something awaken in me again. One lovely lady even makes me up a chart of my post transfer implantation probability. According to her calculations, it may have been too early to test and if implantation had occurred up to eight days after my transfer, then it might still take a few days before the hCG shows up in my urine and, more importantly, is strong enough to register on a home pregnancy test. I quickly researched everything I could find on implantation. It seemed unlikely that the implantation process would take that long. I had a day three transfer, which means that by about day 11, implantation should have occurred. Maybe, just maybe, I did test too soon for the hCG to show up in my urine? Tomorrow I will do another test, but this time I will use first morning urine which works better for low sensitivity tests.

I couldn't think of anything else but getting to the chemist to buy another testing kit. I really should just wait until next week for the blood test, but seeing as I had already put myself through one night of misery, what would it matter if the worst was once again confirmed. I purchased a kit with three highly sensitive tests in it that said they could detect hCG as low as 25. In many early pregnancies, the hCG level starts off low but should double every 31 to 72 hours. As the pregnancy progresses, hCG levels rise and the doubling time increases which indicates a successful pregnancy. The kit even stated that the test could be used up to four days before a missed period. Mine is due in two days—Monday. I parted with another $20 and thought for a brief moment about all the money I have spent on these tests and how I could have bought myself that longed for pair of new season boots by now. I pushed the thought to the back of my head. Shopping for myself depresses me these days. I find it incredibly isolating. Even shopping for an outfit for a new occasion makes me feel like a failure. I don't want to be buying for me anymore, I want to buy for our baby. Sometimes I even wander around the children's section and mentally pick things out. Shopping for myself was like filling the void for the things I really want to be buying. I have often driven home from a shopping trip in tears, but tears are nothing anymore. They are a part of everyday life now. As regular as a morning cup of tea, but without the sugar.

Once I was home, I knew that I would be faced with the evil home pregnancy test dilemma again. I knew I should wait until tomorrow morning before doing another test, but I was incapable of thinking about anything else until I peed on that bloody stick. I locked myself in the bathroom and removed the plastic foil surrounding the test. I didn't need to read the instructions anymore. I took the strip and placed it horizontally in my urine stream for five seconds. Almost immediately a blue dye crossed the test panel window and a line appeared in the control window, indicating that the test had been performed correctly. There are many different types of test on the market, and I have sampled most of them. Still, none of them can offer you 100% accuracy. I sat on the toilet seat and stared at the important window. You should read the results after three minutes. I looked at my watch. Three minutes and no sign of a blue line. My stomach sank in that all too familiar way. I wished I could sink into the toilet and be flushed away. I wiped myself and pulled up my pants. I placed the test strip on the side of the bathroom vanity cabinet. I am so attached to these strips now that I can't bring myself to throwing them away, for fear of missing a positive result. Hence, I have 20 tests lined up alongside my bathroom toiletries. My record is 24. I've gone through months where I've tested every single day, regardless of a negative result. I washed my hands and add the test to my long line of failures.

Year 3, Tuesday 27 February—
Game over

When you jump on the IVF rollercoaster, it's a strapped-in, scary ride. Every move is planned, dates are scrutinised and as the end approaches it becomes a full-time obsession. During the two week wait the daily visits to the clinic are a thing of the past and no-one calls to inform you how your little embryo is snuggling into your uterus. Life, as we know it, now lies within the hands of the gods. Science can only do so much. The power you had during your stimulated cycle is now over. The feeling of being constructive, of actually taking charge and being in control of getting pregnant, has now ended. You must now find something else to occupy your days. That's the scary part. Back to the real fertile world.

If an IVF cycle results in a 'big fat negative', you are advised to have at least one month's break to allow your body to return to normal before embarking on another cycle. What on earth will I occupy the next eight weeks with? More mental affirmations, more acupuncture and more clinging to the hope of maybe just maybe achieving a natural pregnancy. Back to bonking on cue. It doesn't excite me. Nothing does these days. I feel like I'm existing in slow motion, with my real life on pause. I can't make any decisions or plan for the future. Everything is on hold and as much as I'd like to be able to appreciate the good fortune of everything I do have in my life, I can't. Everyday living is clouded. Work is a means to an end—paying for more treatment and sustaining a mortgage. I don't have the passion for anything right now. I hope I won't always feel like this. What if IVF doesn't work? What then? I'm panicked.

My official blood test is just a day away. No sign of my period. As we non-fertiles—and especially we actor/singer non-fertiles—say: "It's not over till the fat lady sings". By that we mean anything's possible until the dreaded period arrives. Pregnant until proven otherwise (PUPO). I however, am not feeling optimistic. I have used up all my positive thinking. Now I have to prepare myself for the worst. The arrival of blood. Another rude smack in the face to erase the eight weeks of praying, routine pricks in the stomach and hope that this would bring us our dream.

A friend suggested I go for a massage to centre my energy and spoil myself. I decided a bit of quiet time would do me good. I didn't expect what was about to happen. I am no longer in control of anything, especially myself.

I don't remember getting to the massage therapy centre. That is a common occurrence these past few days. With so much going on internally, everything else around me fades into the background. I didn't have to wait long until a young girl came out and showed me to the massage table. I opted for a head, neck and shoulder massage. Keep it brief. I put my belongings in a bag under the table and took my place on the table, face down. I was prepared for the pain that engulfed my body. My breasts are so enlarged and tender from the progesterone pessaries that I could not lie flat. My bust has increased at least two cup sizes, another side effect from an IVF cycle. My body believes it is pregnant as I am pumping it with artificial progesterone twice a day until the dreaded blood pregnancy test.

Unexpectedly, tears began to roll down my face and drop into a carefully placed dish under the table that was filled with flowers. It wasn't just the pain in my breasts, it was the pain in my heart. Sadness overwhelmed me and before long my chest began to heave and I couldn't control the emotion that enveloped me. The massage lady kindly left the room and gave me a moment to myself. I didn't know what to say. There was no point in explaining. I gathered my things and left hurriedly without even thinking of paying.

Later. An hour later my dear husband found me on the bathroom floor curled up in a ball. I guess I didn't recognise it at the time, but this was the mental breakdown that I never shared with anyone. When I look back, I think it was my brain shutting down. Shutting out the anxiety and not being able to cope with the finality of never becoming a mum. I knew I was suffering but I didn't acknowledge to what extent. I had channelled the emotion into occupying myself with useless pregnancy facts and HPT obsession. I don't recall how many hours passed or for how long I was on that bathroom floor before Fez found me. I'd erased all memory of getting there. This was life at its lowest.

Year 3, Wednesday 28 February—
Me and my shadow

Today was my scheduled blood pregnancy test and my period was two days late. Perhaps there is still hope. It's this hanging onto hope that is mentally destructive. I am already starved of tears and emotion, what point is there in making myself relive the negative result over and over again. It is an addiction, a drug. I can't let it go.

The two remaining pregnancy tests were neatly tucked underneath the bathroom cabinet, coaxing me to unwrap the foil packaging and read the instruction booklet that I know all too well already. I got out of bed and made my way into the toilet. First morning urine would definitely eliminate any uncertainty of a false negative. I stared at the little plastic stick and placed it in my urine stream for five seconds. Once again, I experienced the familiar head rush and heart palpitations where it felt as if I could never catch my breath. It felt like the world had just stopped. Staring at the results window, I watched as the blue dye made its way over into the control window. Once again a line immediately appeared to indicate the test had been performed correctly. Then it was the three minute wait. Why did I continue to do this to myself?

I placed the stick on the edge of the bath and jumped in the shower. No second guessing myself anymore. This time it was a yes or no answer. Clear as daylight. I managed to take the quickest shower possible and was barely dry before I peered at that stick again. My heart did its usual skip as I caught my breath. There seemed to be a shadow line in the result window. It wasn't a line as such but definitely something I have not seen before. I thrust the stick under the bathroom light. No, I was not imagining it, there was a mysterious dark shadow of a line there. Could it be? It was barely visible but enough to ignite a glimmer of hope. I quickly referred back to the instruction booklet. The words 'evaporation line' jumped out at me from within the tiny black type. An evaporation line occurs when a test has been left for a long time or if there is moisture in the air. Damn, I have just had a shower and the mirrors are full of condensation. I went straight to the internet and research everything I can find about evaporation lines. I read that a line in the window is a positive result regardless. False positives were very rare. Glimmer of hope. I go to the photo page where other people had sent in pictures of their pee sticks. I went to the section clearly marked false positives.

There it was, pages of photos of sticks that look exactly like mine. A shadow of a line, grey in appearance and barely visible. It was a fault in the test. I also read that for a test to be positive, there has to be coloured dye involved. There is a difference between a faint blue line and a faint grey shadow line. Once again, it was all over. I threw the stick away but this time felt strangely empowered. It was the first test I had been able to dispose of immediately. I was not going to be at the mercy of those sticks anymore.

The time has come for me to face the hard truths and come to terms with the fact that not all pee sticks are wrong. In fact they are incredibly accurate. Amidst all the emotions still churning around in me, the hardest task was yet to come. Telling mum. She has been through all of this with me. The excitement of getting 15 eggs, the fertilisation report, the overwhelming elation when the embryo was implanted back into my uterus, the hopes and the fears, but mostly the promise of realising our dream of becoming parents. I picked up the phone knowing I had cried all my tears and dialled mum's number. It was like calling to tell her a part of me had died and I knew she would feel exactly the same way. She reassured me to wait for the blood pregnancy test results—to be sure.

I made my way to the clinic for my official blood pregnancy test by 9.00 am. I made it just in time. I usually get there much earlier than this but no, not today. I had a little bit of control back. Like a slap to the face, the official test is something that is routine for IVF patients, just in case there is a viable pregnancy. Even if a patient gets a period before a blood pregnancy test, the clinic still advises you to come in for your 'official' result. They reassure you that even with bleeding, some women go on to having a positive pregnancy test. It's commonly known as implantation bleeding but it's often a lot lighter than a normal menstrual period. I already knew what my result was—a big, fat negative, but like an obedient patient, I turned up for the test anyway. This time the needle seemed to hurt more. Prior to this, I could put up with the constant pricks in my arm and the bruises that came along with it. The nurse who took my blood had a spring in her step and spoke with optimism.

"So, you've come in for your pregnancy test?" she said with a glint in her eye.

"Yes," I replied. "But I already know the outcome. I peed on a stick last night."

"Oh, I'm so sorry. But we do often see women go on to have positive pregnancy tests even with negative home pregnancy tests", she added. It's almost as if they're programmed to justify why a patient is subjected to this final torture.

"I know," I said, feeling the tears well up in my eyes.

Hello tears. I haven't seen you for a few hours at least. Welcome back.

"I'm not holding out any hope," I say definitively.

The nurse went silent and released the compress from my arm. I felt the blood rush back into my limb.

"Ok, we'll call at around 2.00 pm for your official result. Good luck," she said as I left the sterile bloods room.

Nobody likes to admit to a failure. I made my way out of the clinic to where Fez was waiting for me in the car. I could feel his pain too but it's largely unspoken of. It is unbearable to talk about. Better to just look forward and get on with things. Back to being the strong wife.

I spent the rest of the day at home in a daze. I went about my normal day-to-day duties, checking emails and answering the phone, but things weren't the same. It would be a while before I could function normally again. I have put so much hope on things working out the first time. Everything was all so new and exciting. Once things fail it clouds every future thought of trying again. I don't feel optimistic. I am preparing for failure after failure even though I am assured that my odds get better with every new attempt.

2.45 pm. No call from the clinic. I called to get the official blood pregnancy result. No-one answered so I left a message.

3.30 pm. The clinic finally called me back and apologised for the delay. Apparently there had been a lot of pregnancy tests today. The news was to be as expected. The nurse did her best to put on her sympathy voice and for a moment I felt sorry for her having to deliver the devastating news to so many hopeful women. It was strange that in my ultimate moment of pain, all I could think about was how to make her job easier and reassure her that the news was no surprise and that I was fine. She seemed relieved. Just as I was about to hang up the phone, I asked her if there were any signs of hCG in my blood . . . any indication that implantation had at least tried to occur. There was a pause as she reviewed my results.

"Unfortunately no. No hCG present".

It was a whopping zero. Somehow I felt that if the embryo had at least tried to implant, then perhaps there was some hope to grasp onto for the next cycle but it wasn't to be. Back to square one. Even science can't make the bloody thing stick.

I called Dr Fertility and made an appointment to come in and discuss our plans for our FET. I wanted to get things happening as quickly as possible. But he advised we wait a couple of months to give my body the best possible chance of recovering after all the artificial hormones. Two more long months to wait. I looked at my diary and counted the days. I got onto the internet and looked up success rates for frozen transfers. Variable, but it has worked for some. It seems that there is even less of a success percentage for frozen cycles than fresh. Great. The hope hasn't even begun before it is taken away.*

---

* See Q&A section on an update on the success of frozen embryo transfers

Year 3, Thursday 1 March—
Ticking clock

Today I woke to blood on the bed sheets. Even though it was no surprise, it was still so final. The final curtain call. No standing ovation. No reprise. The end. I got up and placed a towel over the bed sheet and crawled back into bed. I mourned for the loss of our little embryo and for the lost months of hope. Fez was sound asleep beside me. He can sleep through a fire alarm but is oddly kept awake by a ticking clock. I didn't have any more tears but I was sure they'd come back later. It takes so much strength to get to the end, only to realise you have to start all over again.

There are a lot of parallels between my profession and my personal life. I think about the demise of Titanic. How it had started out with so much promise and critical appeal only to fizzle out after only a few weeks on the stage. Being cast in a show like that is a huge achievement in itself. It might take years before I get cast in another major musical. But I will always go for the auditions. The curiosity always gets the better of me, if nothing else. I never give up trying. I spare a thought for all the lives lost on the Titanic. It was uncanny. I guess I could add another life to that loss. I couldn't get back to sleep. Life is full of so many uncertainties.

My mind is already going through all the motions. What month can we start the frozen embryo cycle? I made a mental note to call Dr Fertility again and book in. In the meantime, I will suffer the abdominal cramps in silence. It's much worse than the usual period cramping. I wonder if this is what a miscarriage feels like. This is the reward for all the artificial drugs I have subjected my body to.

I received a message on my mobile phone very early in the morning from my good friend Bec:

"Hi Aunty Debbie, it's Bec here. Give me a call when you get a chance . . . (pause) . . . Aunty Debbie."

Aunty Debbie? But Bec wasn't due for another ten weeks. Surely she couldn't have had the baby? I quickly dialled Bec's phone and heard her answer in a hushed tone. She was in fact in the hospital. What she thought was some mild wind pain had turned out to be the birth of her baby daughter Chelsea Scarlet Blake. I know everything about trying to get pregnant but nothing about premature birth. Could she survive ten weeks early?

Bec and her husband Ian seem to have taken it all in their stride. I guess shock must have set in and I think they're still recovering from the ordeal. But with all the hurdles that will certainly be thrown at them over these next few weeks, they do a great job in concealing any kind of concern or anxiety. Chelsea weighed 3 pounds 13, the upper end of the scale for a baby of 30 weeks gestation. Bec had been having some Braxton Hicks contractions. Luckily for her, and with large thanks to the insight of her obstetrician, Bec was taking steroids just in case those contractions were a sign of early labour. These drugs would help develop the baby's lungs in the event that she was born prematurely. As a result, Chelsea managed to avoid any serious complications. She entered this world a battler and has survived against the odds. There is some inspiration to be gained from that, as well as a sense of relief.

I have come to realise that my friends' actual pregnancies are what I find hardest to deal with. As I processed the early birth of my close friends' baby, I took some pain killers for the cramping and went about scrubbing my blood stained sheets. The last of the lingering reminders of our poor fortune. I hoped Chelsea would be OK.

CHAPTER 9

Getting on with it

"As infertility envelops every inch of your life and soul, it's easy to forget that life continues to go on around you. Every so often, out of the blue, something happens to make you forget your own tunnel vision and snap you back into some sense of the real world."

Year 3, Friday 23 March—
The show must go on

Like any curve ball thrown at you in life, you can never predict when one is about to impact your world. What has been a tragedy over these past few weeks is nothing in comparison to the magnitude of some other people's suffering. It is so easy to get consumed by our own needs and failures, that we fail to recognize just how lucky we really are.

What are the pros and cons of the situation? So what if we couldn't have a family of our own . . . we still have each other. I have a great family and wonderful friends, and we have the freedom and money to travel the world whenever we feel like it.

The week after the official blood test mum said to me that kids aren't everything. I have been thinking about this. How many people have started a family and actually wished they hadn't—secretly fantasising about taking it all back. The loss of independence, freedom and self is something you don't read about in the fertility books.

It's probably a self-defence thing, but I am trying to look at our situation from this point of view. I watch as my girlfriends struggle with their toddlers 24/7, never having a minute to eat their meal or sip their wine. It doesn't look all that appealing to be perfectly honest. But it is a sisterhood. An exclusive club to which one can only gain membership once one has experienced being a mum. For an outsider looking in, what mums do could seem bland compared to a spontaneous, exciting, 'showbiz' life. With my friends, I never really acknowledge their contribution to the 'sisterhood'—I guess I just don't understand it. But they never enquire into my carefree life. I know they are doing their bit for the country—reproducing, nurturing the generations of the future and every other selfless act that comes with being a mother. But I am not a mum (yet), so how could I possibly understand the sacrifice they make.

The weeks are passing and I feel I have stopped counting the days and am beginning to enjoy the daily grind of my life as a self-employed actress/singer. There have been a few auditions around lately and, although I don't feel mentally prepared to attend any of them, they provide a much needed distraction from my infertile world.

I have been offered a job as a walk-in understudy to the incomparable Rhonda Burchmore in a new musical work called Respect: The Musical. I am not in the show exactly, but rather have been hired to learn the show of my own accord and get paid weekly to be on standby in the event that Rhonda goes off sick. The show is about an ageing Broadway diva that takes three young starlets under her wing and teaches them the ropes of show business. I can't believe I'm already being invited to play 'ageing' roles. Geographically, it doesn't make sense. The show is scheduled to do six weeks in each capital city. If there is to be any kind of emergency, it would take me at least four hours to commute by plane to the theatre. However, it is a dream come true. I'll get paid for doing virtually nothing for a year and still be able to live at home and continue with my own life.

Year 3, Thursday 5 April—
Earning a living

I have spent weeks studying the scripts and songs from the comfort of home and, before long, the phone call came to say I had been rostered on for a couple of shows in Brisbane, due to Rhonda's corporate function commitments. This was the call I'd been waiting for, the one that would make me earn my money. As a walk-in understudy, there's not much time for any rehearsals and, having never stepped a foot on the stage, you are really thrown out there with everyone hoping you hit the right marks (spots on the stage—for those who don't know theatre jargon) and make all the right cues. It's highly stressful and is the moment I have to prove to the producers and directors that the weekly wage they have been paying me is money well spent.

Surprisingly, I've been finding it easy to focus on my lines and songs. It is usually quite challenging. Once movement and action is put to a scene, the memory process gets easier because you have something to remember the words by. I have a lot of dialogue to memorise and a lot of experience lately to draw on. One of my songs is a number called "Both Sides Now" by Joni Mitchell. Just reading the lyrics to that song brings up so many emotions.

"I've looked at life from both sides now . . . From win and lose and still somehow . . . It's life's illusions I recall . . . I really don't know life at all . . . But now it's just another show . . . You leave 'em laughing when you go . . . And if you care, don't let them know . . . Don't give yourself away."

The show finishes with another poignant song by Martina McBride called "In My Daughter's Eyes." I've never heard of it until now but somehow I knew this wouldn't be an easy sing either. It would take every bit of professionalism to be able to pull myself together to get some of the words out.

"When she wraps her hand around my finger . . . Oh it puts a smile in my heart . . . Everything becomes a little clearer . . . I realise what life is all about . . . It's hangin' on when your heart has had enough . . . It's giving more when you feel like giving up . . . I've seen the light . . . It's in my daughter's eyes."

Now I will definitely be earning my money.

Year 3, Tuesday 1 May—
Stage Fright

Tonight was my first performance and my nerves were running rampant. Alone in my Brisbane apartment, preparing for the challenge ahead, I was halfway through running my lines in the bathroom when my mobile phone rang. I rushed to the lounge room to pick it up. It was mum. She sounded worried. Attempting to overcome the effect of too much adrenaline coursing through my body, I casually asked her if everything was OK.

"They've found a lump in dad's neck. They think it's malignant. Cancer."

The world stopped. I didn't believe what I was hearing. In just over an hour I was going to be taking to the stage, singing 15 songs I'd never even rehearsed and reciting 50 pages of script in front of a packed house of theatre goers. I couldn't take in what I was hearing. I was stunned. There was silence on the other end of the phone.

"I know you have a show tonight, I didn't want to tell you now but we're seeing the specialist tomorrow and they're going to try and find out where the cancer originated."

I managed to get a few words out: "Are you sure ma? How did this all come about?"

"We found a lump in his neck a few weeks back. We got it checked out and they suggested doing a biopsy there and then. We didn't want to worry you."

Hold on a minute. Mum said they were going to find out where the cancer originated.

"Are you saying this is a secondary cancer mum?"

Mum explained that the original diagnosis was cancer of the parotid (or salivary) gland which is commonly a secondary cancer. They would therefore need to find out where the cancer had started. It is typically from the lung, brain or oral cavity. My mind raced back to when dad was a heavy smoker. He gave up when I was a baby. Was this really happening? I felt so isolated and so far away. I hung up the phone and stared at the clock. I had 15 minutes to make it to the theatre.

Year 3, Wednesday 2 May—
Do good things really happen to those who wait?

I had a mid-morning flight back to Sydney. I spent the early part of the morning staring at the four walls of my apartment, contemplating the news of dad's condition. The results of dad's follow up appointment wouldn't be known until I had landed back in Sydney. I was full of all kinds of emotion. A part of me expected to hear this news at some stage. After all, dad is almost 70. But up until now our whole family has been in good health. I didn't expect the news to have this kind of impact. It has hit me like a blow to the head. The realisation of my unexplained infertility affected me in an entirely different way. Somewhat selfishly, I felt gypped that my kids might not get to know their granddad. I was angry that he probably wouldn't be there to play hide and seek with his grandkids, tortuously tickle them and make up silly nicknames for them. At the same time I am angry at myself for taking his life for granted for so long, and altogether pissed off that the things I want so desperately in life either never happen, or take so bloody long to eventuate that I'm over it by the time they do. I don't want my dad to die. He is my dad. He is the heart and soul of the family. The one man I can always count on to fix things that are impossible for everyone else to fix. He built me my very own ballet bar when I was 10. Now more than ever before, I want to have a baby and I find myself submersed in tears for the loss of what could have been. I have no control over any of it.

A blur has overridden my memory of last night's performance. I got through the show without any major stuff-ups or forgotten lyrics. Just the odd cracked note here and there which comes from too much adrenalin and not letting the voice find its natural rhythm. All in all, it was a bit forced to start with, but that's to be expected—I'd never even run the show in its entirety. There's bound to be room for improvement. Nevertheless, the cast and crew gave me great feedback but it still doesn't stop me from trying to read between the lines and find out what they're really thinking. They were all supportive and complimentary. That's probably all I could cope with right now anyway. I'm drained and there's a lot going on in my head.

It is a week before I am due to fly back to Brisbane again to perform for Rhonda. On arriving home, I received news that they have not been able to find dad's primary cancer so they have scheduled him in for an MRI with another specialist in a few weeks time. In the meantime, we just have to wait. Dad is his usual self, making jokes and reassuring us all that if his time is up, he has had a good life. As usual, I've been pre-occupied with the 'what ifs'. What if we have to move back home, what if mum needs us there for her, what if this is all some awful mistake? Without the doctors having any answers regarding dad's condition, we are all left hanging in limbo. I am fast losing faith in the medical profession. What good are doctors if they themselves don't know what's wrong with you?

Year 3, Friday 11 May—
Brisvegas

I arrived back in Brisbane and stayed on a little longer than expected as Rhonda had taken ill. I've run the show a few times now so I'm gaining confidence and am starting to relax a bit and enjoy myself. It's always an ego boost when the audience laughs or applauds in places that are different from when the main star is on for the role. As an understudy to a celebrity, you don't get to ride off past credits or media exposure. The audience are generally feeling let down that their starring performer is off sick, so they sit on their hands and wait for you to pull out all stops to win them over. I'm on the back foot the moment I walk on stage. These days, big shows don't make an announcement when an understudy performer is on. This is just as well because no performer likes to hear the crowd boo and hiss. Every time I go out on stage, I can only hope that the audience is kind to me and wants to be taken on the journey. If not, they can always kick and scream and demand their money back or tickets for a replacement show.

It is beautiful weather in Brisvegas and I have been enjoying the walk from my apartment to the theatre, it's especially refreshing as the cool night air sets in. Today, as I walked, it crossed my mind that I haven't any idea when my next period is due. It has been four months since we first started IVF and a little over two months since that fateful negative blood test. I really haven't given it much thought since dad's diagnosis. For a brief moment I felt a surge of excitement as I madly tried to calculate when my last period was but not being certain on the exact date. My menstrual cycle has been a little out of whack since the IVF treatment. The fact that I have not been anticipating the arrival of a monthly period is a first in itself. I have known when every single one was due for the past three years! I wondered for a moment if I could be pregnant and in my mind I fantasised about breaking the news to dad, making peace with myself. If only life had the same fairytale endings as in the movies—or in musicals.

Tonight's show went well. Friday night audiences are always up for a good time. At the end of the show I walked out through the theatre foyer and overhear a little old lady remark to her friend:

"Rhonda Burchmore must have dyed her hair blonde. I don't think that was a wig. It really suits her."

That was funny and I chuckled to myself as I walk past them completely unnoticed and made my way home. The shops were still open and it was a beautiful night. I passed a chemist en route and, as if on automatic pilot, I found myself buying a triple pack of pregnancy tests. I made a pact with myself that I wouldn't pee on the stick until morning. At least that would get me through the night.

I am heading to bed with a sense of triumph. I have resisted the urge to pee on a stick and, for the first time in years, don't know when my period is due. In some strange way, I feel in control again.

Year 3, Saturday 12 May— *Confirmation*

I woke up to the sun peeking through my bedroom's wooden venetian blinds. I lay in bed for a moment, drifting back to sleep until my brain kicked in and, like a small child on Christmas morning, I remembered the pregnancy tests sitting on the bathroom cabinet. My heart skipped a beat. I was somewhat reluctant to take the test as I was enjoying my new-found power and hope. I casually got myself out of bed and walked into the living room to switch on my mobile phone. It was way too early to have messages, but any distraction would be appreciated. Then, as I could not physically hold it in any longer, I retreated to the bathroom and succumbed to the all too familiar pregnancy test kit. If my calculations were correct, my period could be as much as one week late but I can't be sure. I tore open the plastic wrapping and proceeded to pee on the stick for 10 seconds. Done. Nothing to do now but wait.

I didn't time it, if that blue line was going to come up it would do so immediately. I placed the stick on a flat surface and washed my hands before glancing back at it. My heart stopped. No way. There were two blue lines. I fell to my knees right onto the cold bathroom tiles and sobbed, clutching the stick like it was my lifeline. This was it. I'd done it. Shaking uncontrollably I reached for my phone and dialled Fez's number. It was only 8.30 am in the morning. The phone rang a couple of times before a very weary Fez answered. I didn't wait for him to speak.

"Honey, can you do me a favour?"

"Deb, its 8.30 am in the morning."

"Yes I know but I really need you to do something for me," I said, trying not to ruin the surprise. "Can you go outside onto the balcony and look up at the sky."

Reluctantly Fez obliged. I told him the news.

"You're going to be a daddy," I whispered, I still couldn't grasp the concept of what was happening.

"What?"

"I'm pregnant. My period is late but I didn't remember 'til yesterday so I took a test this morning. It's positive. I can't believe it and it happened naturally honey. Oh my God, I wish you were here with me."

There wasn't any response from the other end of the phone.

"Fez. I said I'm pregnant!"

"Are you sure babe?" he asked me in a calm, monotone voice. I wanted to scream at him. This was our moment and he was dismissing it like I'd just told him we are out of milk.

"Fez there are two blue lines. I'm not imagining it this time. It came up straight away. Aren't you happy?"

"I'm just cautious Deb. You know how unreliable these things can be. Just take it easy and wait until you can get to the doctors for a blood test."

This is not the reaction I had dreamed about for years. I had waited a long time for those two bloody blue lines and now I wanted to shout it from the top of the apartment block.

"OK, I'll try and book in to the doctors this morning. That way we'll know for sure daddy." I was chuckling now.

"Look, promise me you won't tell anyone until you get confirmation from the docs. Not even your mum—OK? Are you sure there are two lines?"

I glanced back at the pregnancy test. There it was, exactly where I had left it on the bathroom cabinet when I picked up the phone to call Fez. I put it up to the light and felt the blood drain from my veins. The line had disappeared. There was only one blue line. What had happened? I knew I didn't imagine it. I shook that damn test, I ripped it apart for proof of that blue line. Nothing. Shaking, I got another out of the packet and peed again. Nothing. Zilch. I fell to my knees again and howled into the cold bathroom tiles.

Why me? I didn't imagine it. That line was there. Clear as day. I had been pregnant for five minutes.

~

Later I went to the local pathology centre and demanded a blood pregnancy test. I pleaded with the doctor to rush the results of my test through and to call me before the day was over. I had another show later tonight but couldn't concentrate on anything until I got those results. Half an hour before the clinic closed I called to get my results. The receptionist was supposed to call me. I am put on hold as they retrieved my file. It felt like an eternity.

"Mrs Krizak, do you mind calling back in half an hour, we don't seem to have the results in as yet."

"Sure. But I really need to get the results today."

I hang up the phone. I am desperately clinging onto anything. A blue line is a blue line I keep telling myself, I didn't imagine it. I'm not going crazy.

When I called back, the results were in. Negative. I asked if there had been any trace of hCG in the blood reading. There wasn't. It is zero which means a pregnancy never even existed. The hardest part of all was yet to come—calling Fez and taking it all back. My phone rang. It was mum. She has an intuitive way of knowing when something is wrong. I told her the news. Mum being her beautiful self listened with compassion and shared my grief. I could tell she felt every bit of pain. My sobs subsided and my thoughts turned to dad. I asked if there had been any more news.

"Yes darling. He's in the clear. The lump disappeared overnight and the doctors have admitted it was a misdiagnosis. They are completely baffled by it," mum said in a calm, controlled manner.

"What? You're saying he doesn't have cancer . . . That it's gone?"

"Yes dear. There never was any cancer. They got it wrong."

And for the third time today I fell to my knees. This time I cried tears of joy and relief. Miracles do happen. If that was all the luck I had in my life, then I was happy to take it right there and then.

As infertility envelops every inch of your life and soul, it's easy to forget that life continues to go on around you. Every so often, out of the blue, something happens to make you forget your own tunnel vision and snap you back into some sense of the real world. Sometimes these occurrences are like a breath of fresh air, even if it isn't always good news.

I have a renewed vigour for tonight's show. There is the weight of disappointment on my back but I also appreciate the value of life. Of living. Now. Living like life can be taken away from you at any moment. Somehow the picture's a bit clearer. The tears stream down my face in "Both Sides Now" and I have the audience in the palm of my hand—

with me every step of the way. I change out of my costume and notice some spotting on my G string. My period has arrived.

Year 3, Wednesday 16 May— *Maternity Ward*

We decided to make the trip to Adelaide to see baby Chelsea. She was still in intensive care but doing exceptionally well despite the odds. Fez and I agreed to visit Chelsea in hospital. I was feeling cautious. I didn't know if my emotions would hold out, especially being in a maternity ward watching new young mums basking in the weary glory of first time motherhood. Nevertheless, we made the trip to Ashford Hospital and watch as both Ian and Bec picked up their tiny new baby and gave her a bath. She was so delicate. I glanced around the intensive care unit and saw many babies hooked up to the tubes and wires that were monitoring their every breath. Mothers sat with their babies gently rocking them and inhaling that sweet smell of new young life. I was instantly drawn to a lady who sat quietly holding a hand each of her newborn twins.

I felt compelled to walk over to her and ask how she was doing. The twins were born six weeks early and the concern shows on her face. I have never thought about worries like these. I always thought getting pregnant was the be all and end all, but even throughout pregnancy things can go wrong and I've never even contemplated complications once a baby had been born. I guess my own mother was right. The worry never stops from the minute they're born. Yet that seems so far down the track for me. If there is a light at the end of the tunnel, I am still completely immersed in pitch black.

We left the hospital after spending half an hour with Chelsea. It is difficult for Bec to visit and leave her daughter day after day. With any luck she will be able to take her home in four weeks time. I know all too well that four weeks can feel like an eternity. I gave her a hug and out of the corner of my eye I caught Fez wiping away a tear. This was a turning point for us. The ever optimistic Fez was getting a glimpse into my tortured world and, during that brief half hour, realisation hit him that he may never get to hold his own child in his arms. It was heartbreaking.

Year 3, Sunday 20 May— *Baby Shower*

We stayed a few extra days in Adelaide as it was Bec's baby shower today. I mustered all my strength and dignity to organise it—the invitations, party games, food and of course cocktails. It was the first baby shower I have ever attended where the baby was already born and the mum could enjoy a few drinks. It turned out to be a wonderful day and I actually managed to enjoy myself . . . even the part when Bec opened all those tiny baby gifts to the echoes of all her girlfriends oohing and aahing. I am genuinely happy for her and Ian, even though I am not yet wearing that red polka dot dress. I started to think about our next IVF cycle. I must get onto that as soon as we return home.

Year 3, Tuesday 22 May—
The big 'O'

We arrived back in Sydney and Fez and I have received an invite to join friends up in the Blue Mountains for the weekend. After a busy few months, we thought it would be nice to get away for some long overdue rest and relaxation. I couldn't wait. We also decided that upon returning to Sydney we would try again with a FET. We will thaw one of our frozen embryos and have it transferred, the same way as a fresh cycle but without all the stimulation drugs.

We have two frozen embryos and, as soon as I ovulate, the embryo will be thawed and inserted through a catheter. Timing is crucial. On a typical 28 day cycle, ovulation could occur anywhere from day 10 to day 16. In order to be in line with my body's natural ovulation cycle, daily blood tests will be taken to see when my hormones surge. This will enable the frozen embryo to be put back three days later (at the same stage it at which it was frozen), when my endometrium is fully ripe for implantation.

I called the clinic and arranged to start with the FET. The nurse asked me how far I am in my monthly cycle and I told her my last period was close to ten or eleven days ago. She told me to come in for a blood test immediately so we could determine if this month was a viable time to commence.

I made my way to the clinic and had my blood taken. It was strange walking back into this place after being gone for a few months. It felt like stepping back in time. I hoped that this time would be a more positive experience though. The purpose for the blood test was to check to see whether my hormones had surged, indicating that I was ovulating. I was pretty certain I was getting close. All the physical signs are here—mucus discharge, increased sex drive, craving for salt. I was anticipating having the transfer on the Tuesday after our weekend away. I'd have ovulated by then surely.

The nurse from the clinic called to tell me that my hormone levels were still low and that no surge had been detected as yet. I made an appointment to go in again tomorrow, and every day if necessary until my hormone surge was detected. The good news was, we were set for an FET this month and everything was on track. It was just a waiting game now until I ovulated.

Year 3, Friday 25 May—
14 days and counting . . .

My arms are beginning to look like pin cushions and the bruises from all the blood tests make me look like a drug addict. The longer this goes on, the more chance of us having to cut short our getaway. If I get the call to say I've ovulated today, then I'll have to be back at the hospital first thing Monday morning for my transfer which means leaving our holiday accommodation on the Sunday to be back in time. I am beginning to get anxious again. I got to the clinic first thing for another blood test and listened to the all too familiar instructions. I would receive a call this afternoon to inform me of my results. Keep the weekend free. Be prepared for transfer anywhere up to 36 hours after ovulation. We put off leaving for our getaway until the following morning. Just in case we needed to have another blood test before setting off. I hate always being in limbo.

Year 3, Tuesday 29 May—
Money for nothing

It is day 18 and I finally ovulated. We cancelled our trip to the mountains as my hormone readings were showing that I wasn't even close to ovulating. Hence, we would have had to travel back to the city again on the Sunday morning. Pointless really. So we bailed. Another sacrifice for a 'maybe'. I was asked to come into the clinic to collect the hormone pessaries that I would need to insert over the next five days leading up to the transfer.

As well as picking up the drugs, the final bill for the FET had to be paid. They make sure you pay before the transfer because on occasions, the embryo doesn't survive the thaw and there is nothing to implant, leaving patients with a whole lot of emotional fallout. As I handed over my money, I felt desperate. This wasn't an emotion I expected to surface. Paying for a baby, for a chance of having life grow inside of me. The God-given right for womankind and I was having to pay for it. I was depressed and ashamed. Handing over my credit card in exchange for a baby. I haven't been counting exactly, but I'd estimated we've paid in excess of eight thousand dollars so far. How had it all come to this?

I have to wait two whole days now until the day of transfer which has been scheduled for Friday 1 June. That's provided our embryo survives the thawing process and we have something to transfer.

Just after dinner tonight I received a call from the clinic. The embryologist has called me personally to inform me that the first embryo they thawed did not survive. In simple terms, the tiny embryo did not have enough battery power to grow any more cells. The embryologist was very matter of fact about the process and tried to encourage me by saying they have already proceeded to thaw our remaining embryo and that I should turn up to the clinic at the scheduled time of 10.00 am Friday morning.

I was feeling a mixture of strange emotions. Happy that a transfer time had been established and good to have the knowledge of what's happening next, but nervous about the outcome. In anticipation, I packed my bag for the day surgery, there would be no anaesthetic this time and we would probably only be at the clinic for an hour in total. I decided to have an early night. I was brushing my teeth in my pyjamas and the all too familiar tears started to fall. I felt a real sadness and loss for our little embryo. I didn't realise I had become so attached to these microscopic cells of promise. I grieved momentarily for the child and put myself to bed. Despite the FET odds, maybe this would be third time lucky. Fingers, toes and everything crossed.

Year 3, Friday 1 June—
Another day at the office

I awoke after a rather restless night in anticipation of the day's events ahead. There was still that desperate pit of sadness deep within me as I processed Tuesday's phone call once again in my head. I wondered what that child would have looked like. I wondered if it would have survived if we hadn't made the decision to freeze it. Had I killed my child? The guilt that came with all of this was overwhelming. But there is nothing natural about the IVF process and I have to accept that a natural pregnancy progression without human or scientific intervention is not a luxury we are to be afforded.

We arrived at the day surgery with enough time to fill out our transfer forms, waiving all legal rights and signing off on the fact that we had the same likelihood of pregnancy as winning lotto. Reassuring. Fez and I were taken into a small room which consisted of a TV monitor and a large black chair with the all too familiar leg stirrups. It felt like a waiting room. Within minutes Dr Fertility made his way into the room to greet us and put on his plastic gloves. I wasn't feeling as comfortable at seeing him as I was the first time. Something bothered me about him now. I had a gut feeling that he was used to telling patients what they wanted to hear but there was no pulling the wool over my eyes this time. I knew what I was up against.

"Now you've spoken to the embryologist?"

"No, not yet," we both responded in unison.

There was a pause and Dr Fertility left the room before returning with the embryologist. She was a small, well spoken Asian lady holding a clipboard and sporting an ID tag. Once I confirmed my name and the procedure I was about to undergo, she explained to us that our remaining embryo had thawed sufficiently but had only continued to grow by one cell. At this stage in the game, our little embryo should have been eight cells. If not, then it should have been at least an even number of cells. Ours was five cells with a significant amount of fragmentation, which means a percentage of the embryo had broken off into pieces during cell division. From my understanding, this wasn't a good sign. For an embryo to be of good quality, it needs good clean cell division with minimal fragmentation. The pit in the bottom of my stomach fell through my spine. Why hadn't anyone called me? Why had I come in, believing I was to have a transfer when there is nothing to transfer but a good-for-nothing five-cell . . .

"I don't anticipate a successful pregnancy from this transfer, but we have seen miracles occur before so we're going to give it a go and proceed with the transfer in the hope that the embryo will thrive better in the natural environment of your womb."

I was speechless. Everything was going in slow motion. They showed us our little five cell on the TV monitor and within moments I had had the transfer. I got up straight away and put my jeans on.

"Let's get out of here," I said to Fez as we whisked our way past the receptionist. I vaguely heard her shouting out "Good luck" after us as the door shut behind us.

As we drove home the questions flooded in. Why weren't we informed about the embryo? Why did the transfer still go ahead? This was additional emotional fallout I didn't need. False hope. I hated the feeling of being kept in the dark.

I didn't even give that embryo inside me another thought. Positive thinking had long fallen by the wayside. It was a numbers game now and if the numbers weren't right then it would be another failure.

We decided to invite some friends around for dinner instead of being alone. I was going to have a few drinks—even though I was considered technically pregnant in a one-in-a-million-chance kind of way. Our friends Greg and Caz joined us and we planned a nice casual dinner—with copious amounts of champagne. I decided to make my favourite champagne and guava cocktail to greet our friends. We chinked our glasses on their arrival. Our friend Caz lowered her glass and discreetly placed it on the breakfast bar.

Greg and Caz met quite late in life and fell pregnant in their forties. Caz is now 42. I felt the bubble of despair rise up inside of me as I anticipated the announcement. Caz was looking a little sheepish. Greg was quick to defend his wife's mood, explaining she was not feeling too well.

"Here we go again," I thought. "Two out of three . . . not drinking, feeling ill." I am a master detective when it came to sniffing out pregnancies. "Please don't let it be the case." I tried not to think about it and engaged in conversation.

We all sat at the table and I served entrée. Caz had still not touched her champagne and the boys were having a good old catch up. I sat down next to Caz and sensed her uneasiness. "Caz, you're pregnant again aren't you?"

She looked up at me while twirling her champagne glass and obviously didn't know what to say. "Oh Deb, I didn't want to say anything. It's only very early days and I haven't even been to the doctor yet. I'm sorry I didn't want to tell you. I know what you've been going through."

Caz was so sincere and beautiful. I was happy for her. It's just that I was desperately unhappy for myself. That's life. It doesn't stop around you. In cruel twists of fate, life seems to challenge you and throw you these curveballs whenever you seem to be at breaking point.

"Was it planned?"

"Yes. We thought we better get a move on now I'm 42. We thought we might have problems, given my age, and it didn't happen immediately." Greg and Caz already had a daughter who is almost two. "How long were you trying?" I asked. "It took us three months to fall," she said.

It was the answer I was dreading. Luckily I was distracted by the overflowing boiling water on the stovetop. Three whole months. Would you believe it? I took another gulp of champagne.

Year 3, Friday 15 June—
Education is power

It was no great shock to get my period exactly 14 days after our five cell tragedy. During this past fortnight I have felt every emotion possible. Anger was the one that was more prevalent this time around. Anger at feeling conned by the clinic and anger that I have not taken more initiative to be in control of my procedures. I always waited for the phone to ring. From now on, I'll be doing the ringing.

Some good has managed to come out of our five cell experience. Fez and I have been talking about changing clinics. We don't have any more frozen embryos and our only option is to undergo another fully stimulated drug cycle of IVF. After our recent treatment, I am not convinced we chose the best clinic. I have been researching options on the internet and have been shocked at what I've discovered. Yes, I had previously researched everything about the processes involved with IVF but never once did I consider researching the actual clinics themselves or the differences between them.

The clinic we had chosen supported day three transfers, and had never once mentioned a procedure called blastocyst transfers which is where embryos are allowed to develop to a day five stage before being transferred to a patient. I am an internet research junkie. I can't believe I didn't check the clinic out online and compare their success rates. I have now delved into the various laboratory techniques clinics used to develop the embryos. I've also research which clinics have the highest live birth rate for women of my age and locate a fabulous clinic right under our noses.

Despite the cynicism I have developed about the business of fertility treatment, I am willing to give this new clinic a try—even though it is more expensive than our current clinic. Fez and I have decided that if we are going to dedicate this year to IVF, then we don't want to waste any more time and money with second rate operators. We will pay the price and book ourselves in for an appointment as soon as possible. The clinic is Genea (formerly Sydney IVF) and we have to wait before we can get to see someone. Everyday seems like an eternity.

I continue researching Genea's services online and start finding glowing reports from all around the world. I find they are at the forefront of day 5 embryo culture. There were many stories of success for couples who had been unsuccessful elsewhere.

I found myself liberated by all this new information and talked it over with Fez. We will need to make a financial plan. Our business pretty much takes care of itself and brings in enough income to pay the mortgage and bills. We're at the stage now where many of our acts are sought after and the bookings come to us, rather than us having to chase work all the time. Still, there are always quiet times where cash flow gets a bit low and momentary panic sets in. Somehow we always manage to get through. I'll take a job teaching dance, giving singing lessons, or stepping up my commercial work. There is always a way around the showbiz slump. Any down time we get we use to create new acts and this is primarily what Fez does. However, having to come up with the money for treatment up front, one treatment cycle will just about clean us up of all of our disposable cash and savings. Not to mention if it doesn't work the first time.

There's no question that we have to do this and Fez agrees. We have to try everything, no matter the cost. We'd never forgive ourselves if we didn't. I made a few calls to our bank and discovered that we are in advance on our mortgage payments and are able to redraw the surplus. It would take seven working days and we would have ten thousand dollars available to us. It is just meant to be.

I also started researching the benefits of Chinese herbs in conjunction with IVF. I saw an article on one of my internet forums that spoke about the relationship between Chinese herbs and IVF success. I Googled as much as I could find out and came across a Chinese Herbalist not far from me and arranged an appointment. She claims to have success helping women achieve pregnancy after numerous failed fertility treatments, miscarriages and hormonal imbalances. I am on a quest to give this new start the best possible opportunity.

Year 3, Thursday 21 June—
Herbalicious?

I arrived at the Chinese doctor early enough to be able to have a look over her rooms and read all the messages of support from other like-minded patients. It was great to read so many positive stories of success. Some of them were truly inspiring. I felt uplifted and positive and in charge of my infertility. I trust my instincts.

When I first met my Chinese doctor, I was astounded at just how flustered she appeared to be. She has no idea if I am a new or existing client (which probably doesn't say much for her regulars). I got the distinct feeling I was talking to a very stressed and busy lady. She spoke so fast that I had to concentrate intently on every word, her thick Chinese accent adding to my difficulty deciphering what she is saying. She asked me a series of questions and began to draw a monthly planner of herbs to aid in conception and marked down what she referred to as the 'sticky' time. The sticky time is her phrase for the implantation process. This is when most pregnancies fail, especially in IVF. She wrote out what herbs I was to take, as well as recommending a course of acupuncture with her. (I gave up on my earlier acupuncture when the first cycle failed.)

As I sit here, I can't help feeling as if I am part of some very clever production line of infertile women, buying and taking herbs that taste disgusting, lined up to be subjected to countless needles. Nevertheless, the results will speak for themselves and, other than costing $350 a visit, what do I have to lose? I bought the herbs and promised to make a follow up appointment in a few weeks. I wonder if she'll remember me by then.

CHAPTER 10

A strange twist of fate

"A person often meets his destiny on the road he took to avoid it."—JEAN DE LA FONTAINE

Year 3, Saturday 23 June—
One Last hurrah

It has been years since Fez and I have been on an overseas holiday. So we've decided to take everyone's 'words of wisdom' literally, and take a holiday away from all the pressures of IVF. It will do us the world of good to get away for four weeks, travel around without a care in the world, just to feel young again. On a whim we booked a trip to see our family in the UK and then do a whirlwind tour of Italy, Greece and Santorini. There is so much beauty to discover.

Fez has taken to planning the itinerary like a duck to water. It is a welcome distraction. We booked our tickets to depart Sydney in two weeks time. It has all happened so fast. It feels great to get some spontaneity back into our lives, where the only thing we really had to plan for was our relaxation and enjoyment. This feels new. I'm excited. We paid for the holiday on credit, just in case we need our cash for the unthinkable—a third round of IVF.

Year 3, Saturday 7 July—
Take off

We left Sydney with the added excitement that mum and dad were now going to meet us in Singapore and join us for the UK leg of our trip. We planned to catch a flight together to Heathrow.

We landed in Singapore and met mum and dad in the hotel lobby. We spent the evening roaming the markets and cramming in as many tourist opportunities as we possibly could. It was so fabulous sipping on a Singapore Sling in Singapore and getting lost in the throngs of tourists with mum, dad and Fez. I felt so at ease.

Year 3, Sunday 8 July—
Other side of the world

It was a long flight and my feet are swollen. I really should have thought about doing those exercises they tell you about in the in-flight magazine. Instead, I grabbed another trashy tabloid magazine and called the flight attendant to ask for another glass of wine. I'm on holidays. I'm allowed to.

There were quite a few families travelling with young children. A lady was walking her toddler up and down the plane aisles. She must have caught me smiling at her as she passed by my seat.

"How old is he?" mum asked.

"Oh, he's 15 months old now. My miracle baby."

Miracle baby. A total stranger stopped by our seat to proclaim her child a miracle baby. Everything went into slow motion. All the pieces fit together. This meeting felt like something more than just a coincidence. I got tingles up my spine as I waited for her to explain.

"We had him on our fourth IVF attempt. They'd just about given up hope for us and then he came along and proved them all wrong."

We both sat and listened to this gorgeous woman tell of her story of despair, hope and finally success. It was obvious she was deeply moved by her experience. I was completely shellshocked that she was just offering this information so freely, and to total strangers. There was a substantial pause before my mum blurted out my story in return. The woman was overcome with emotion and leaned over to give me a hug. It was as if this lady had been sent to us from a heavenly source. She told me to hang in there and to never give up hope. She said she almost did and, as she hugged her young son, tears fell from her eyes. Her words were more poignant than I could ever imagine. I didn't get her name nor did I see her again on the flight but I'll never forget her generosity and the sheer randomness of it all.

Year 3, Monday 16 July—
Eye in the sky

Upon arriving in the UK, the four of us spent a few days in the heart of London before heading off to see some relatives in the English countryside. Although Fez was terribly afraid of heights, he agreed to come on the London Eye with us and see the sights of London from hundreds of metres above ground level. We queued for hours to get on, just so Fez could sit terrified as we are suspended above ground. I began to feel nauseous in sympathy with him, the kind of feeling you get when you haven't eaten for a while but you know you couldn't possibly eat. My mind wandered back to the Deb I'd left behind. What if I was feeling sick for real? I could talk myself into any pregnancy symptom. I must have done that a thousand times. No, this was real. I was feeling sick and it wasn't from the height. I had no idea when my period was due, I was on holiday for God's sake! I deliberately left all that behind when I stepped on the plane back in Sydney. Problem is, as I cast my mind back and started doing the maths, I realised I must have been at least three days late. Having said that, my cycle hadn't been the usual 28 days since I started treatment. No—it must be all the travel and the changes in time zones. Almost certainly.

When we finished on the London Eye we stopped for a quick coffee before finding our way back to our hotel. I was still nauseous and the smell of coffee was quite offensive. My God, could I be? Maybe it is the herbs I'm taking? Yes, I've been subjecting myself to these muddy, vile-tasting concoctions since I parted with my $350 at the Chinese doctors. I couldn't justify the spending without following through, so I've been holding my nose every morning and night and downing as much of the stuff as I can physically stomach. I was momentarily distracted . . . did I really want to set myself up for another disappointment—especially whilst I was on holiday? No, I couldn't go there, not now. To satisfy my old self, I bought a pregnancy test kit on the walk back to our hotel. But I decided I wouldn't use it until Saturday. That way I would be almost certainly over a week late and if I hadn't got my period by then I could justify peeing on another one of those damn sticks, even if I was on the other side of the world. Knowing me, my period would arrive overnight and this would be nothing but another jab in the guts to remind me of home. God damn it.

Year 3, Tuesday 17 July—
A new day and a new life

Morning rolled around and I couldn't sleep in. I reached down to feel for the all too familiar sensation of dry blood on my inner thighs but felt nothing. The familiar stirrings of excitement rose up within me. Fez was still asleep and I had no idea what time it was. It didn't sound like anyone else was up. I reached for the pregnancy kit and read the instructions.

"Detects a positive pregnancy up to five days before your period is due," it proclaimed.

My mind ran through all the possible scenarios. Today we were due to travel to my cousin's place which was about four hours away. I knew I would spend the whole time haunted by an unopened test. If I got it out of the way now and the test came back negative, at least I could just get back on with enjoying our holiday. I didn't want to waste another day with those wretched 'what ifs'. I justified giving in to the test earlier than I'd mentally planned to.

I got up out of bed, shuddering at the cold, and made my way to the upstairs bathroom alongside my parents' room. The test was opened and primed. I peed on the stick for five seconds, replace the cap and pulled up my pyjamas. Time stopped. It came up immediately. Two bright red lines. Before I even had time to put the test down. This was it. I was pregnant. I was pregnant naturally! I had to go to the other side of the world to finally see those two lines but it was the best thing ever. I made sure I was not dreaming. I shut my eyes and opened them after a few seconds. Yes, there were indeed two very strong red lines on that test. Oh my God. I was in shock.

I stopped shaking enough to go and share the news with Fez. This was a strong, definite line. No doubt about it. No squinting required. No ripping the test apart. Just two strong red lines. I couldn't believe this was happening. God knows Fez and I had had enough false alarms over the years, but this was the first time we'd got there. We were pregnant! From my calculations, I was about five weeks pregnant. I walked into the bedroom where Fez was still sound asleep. I tried whispering "Fez" in an immediate tone that I hoped would wake him. No luck. I sat on the edge of the bed and glanced down at the stick again. I couldn't afford to be wrong after what I had put him through in Brisbane. OK, here goes. I shook him until he woke in a stupor and bolted upright. I normally wouldn't do that unless a fire alarm had sounded or I'd heard an odd noise in the night.

"Shh, it's OK, everything's OK," I whispered, trying to soften the alarm of waking him so abruptly.

"Wha . . . What time is it?" he blurted out "Early. It's not time to get up yet." It was still dark outside and I didn't want to tell him the news until he was fully awake.

Before he had time to fall back to sleep, I waved the test in front of his face and showed him the two positive lines. "What's it mean? I thought you were going to wait until Saturday . . . Are you OK?"

He was still half asleep. "I couldn't wait so I took the test when I woke up and I didn't even have to wait for the lines on the test to appear. They came up straight away! It must be a strong pregnancy," I told him.

Fez leaned over and gave me a hug. I could feel some reservations but nothing could taint this moment of bliss for me. "Oh baby, see I told you it would happen. Just be careful not to tell anyone yet OK? It's still early," Fez said.

I crawled back into bed beside Fez but there was no way I could fall back to sleep. I snuggled into Fez's warm chest and processed the enormity of this moment. The beginning of so much. The end of the struggle.

When Fez had fallen back to sleep, I was bursting to tell someone else. It was still only 5.30 am, but I made my way into my parent's room with the stick clasped firmly in my hand and climbed into bed with mum. She woke up in a fluster, thinking something must have been up.

"Hello grandma," I announced.

Dad was still asleep, oblivious to my entering the room. I pulled the stick out and opened the curtain to show mum. We cuddled and cried and thanked God . . . oh and those magic herbs. The Chinese doctor's herbs had worked. I desperately wanted to phone her. It was a revelation and I couldn't wait to share it with the rest of the world. But first, I had to wake dad. It didn't take long as I heard him stirring from all the excited chatter beside him. We shared the news with dad. I wasn't sure if it was mum or me that actually broke the news. Regardless, it was the moment that sealed the deal. Finally telling dad he would be a grandad and knowing that I would do everything in my power to make sure this child got to spend as much time getting to know my wonderful, selfless parents. I felt complete.

There is something incredibly empowering about carrying around a little secret. When you finally fall pregnant after so long, you feel as if you have won the lottery. There was no way I could contain my excitement. After breakfast I told my Uncle and Aunty who we are staying with. We decided we will tell immediate family as well as my two best friends Bec and Suzy back home. I began by texting my brothers in Australia. The messages of congratulations were coming in thick and fast. Everyone was so genuinely happy for us. I'd dreamt of this moment for so long. With the announcement came a rush of excitement as well as the realisation that we hadn't got much further than five weeks in the pregnancy and waiting the full 12 weeks before telling anyone else would be yet another huge challenge.

We set out on the long car journey to my cousin's place in the country. I made a quick stop at the chemist before heading off and armed myself with a supply of home pregnancy tests. It would be a long four days if I couldn't get that rush of peeing on another stick to see those two red lines. After spending almost the equivalent of fifty dollars on tests, I settled in for my first road trip as a newly pregnant mum-to-be, all the while clutching that earlier pregnancy test. The lines had gotten so dark, they looked black. That could only mean I was producing strong pregnancy hormones and maybe I was a little further along than I thought.

We arrived at my cousin John's house and I had a full bladder. I headed straight to the toilet with a new test in my handbag. I'd bought a couple of different brands just to compare lines and how quickly they emerged. The one I was about to use detected pregnancy five days after a missed period. This should give me more idea about how far along I am.

The test was smaller and the dye was blue this time. A simple straight line was to be read as negative and if a cross appeared then the test was positive. Hmmm . . . tricky. I waited for the recommended two minutes before I looked at the test. The result came up slowly, not as fast as I would have thought given the response on my earlier test. After ten minutes, a cross appeared but the line across was fainter. I didn't get the same rush I got earlier in the day. But a cross is a cross and if read within the stated timeframe it meant I was pregnant so all was confirmed.

I managed to immerse myself in family business, drifting in and out of conversations as I let my mind wander to this newly pregnant me phase. It felt so good to have the infertility monkey off my back and all the hardships of the past seemed just a distant memory. I felt reborn.

It had been a wonderful day in the countryside, having lunch in a quaint English pub and reminiscing about past family catch-ups. We decided to get an early night and rest up before tomorrow. Dad had already taken himself off to bed as he wasn't feeling well and was trying to ward off the beginnings of what could be a flu. It was the end of a great day and the start of the most remarkable journey of my life.

During the night I woke up in a sweat and decided to get up and go to the toilet. Not wanting to pass up another full bladder opportunity, I quietly opened another test and took another test. I decided to go back to the original type. I thought nothing as I waited the designated test time for the lines to appear. Sure enough two red lines came up almost immediately and I breathed a sigh of relief. I got a drink of water, washed my hands and peered at the test again before making my way back to bed. Funnily enough, the control line was as dark as the first test I took but the actual pregnancy line was considerably fainter. From all accounts I'd read on the internet blog sites, test lines are supposed to get darker every 48 hours or so to support the increasing hormone levels. Maybe the dyes used in the tests are all different, so I made a pact to do some research on the internet first thing in the morning.

Year 3, Wednesday 18 July—
Teetering on a line

Morning came and I woke with a headache and a sharp pain in my back. The bed wasn't particularly easy on my back, but I never usually take well to different mattresses. I needed to find out what pain relief I could take whilst being pregnant so I logged on to the net and went about looking up home pregnancy test sites. It's amazing what you can find on the net. Sometimes however, ignorance is bliss. I found numerous pictures of the brand of test I had used and they all agreed that the dye can differ for each test and that you can't use the test to tell you 'how pregnant' you are. Surely though, the more hormone present in the urine, the darker the line right? Well according to some other women's pictures of their positively pregnant results, there is a considerable difference in darkness a few days later. I am amazed that women will line up all their tests and sign them with the date and time on them. There are clearly quite a few of us neurotic women out there!

I retrieved my two sticks from my pyjama pocket and went about analysing them under the light. Just when I thought I was over all this second guessing, I was back on it again. My second test is clearly lighter in appearance. It had been about 38 hours between tests, perhaps not long enough for a marked improvement. But why did the line appear fainter than the first test taken? Doubt was back in my head and my head was pounding.

Year 3, Friday 20 July—
Man Flu

I have spent the last two days peeing on a stick at every possible opportunity until I exhausted my total supply. None have given me the result I was hoping to see. But all of them say I am indeed pregnant. That is good enough for me. But I am still feeling a bit dubious. Dad has come down with a full blown flu and we haven't seen him for the last two days. He isn't eating and is sweating it out in bed with a high temperature and the chills. We are pretty much laying low and waiting for him to get better so we can keep travelling.

Year 3, Sunday 22 July—
Paralysed

We have all caught the bug and we are all in a miserable state. I can barely walk. Today I was so crippled with a back spasm as a result of the flu, that I asked Fez to take me to the local hospital. The hospital confirmed that my temperature was high and that I did have a fever. I then asked them to confirm whether I was pregnant or not so I knew what pain relief I was able to take. The doctor took a simple urine test and came back with the results.

"Well you are pregnant and in the very early stages Mrs Krizak," he said tentatively as if this wasn't possibly the best news ever.

"That's OK. We've been trying for a while so we're happy about it." The doctor looked relieved. "Can I just ask how far along do you think I am," I asked the doctor meekly.

"Very early stages. You only just got a positive reading on our pregnancy test. I had to get another doctor to verify it as the line was so faint, but definitely there so, yes, you're most certainly pregnant."

The smile dissolved off my face. I should have been almost six weeks by now. Far along enough to get a stronger reading than a barely visible line.

"How sensitive is the test you use doctor?"

"We use a standard testing system in the hospital. The test picks up an hCG reading of about 50 which you'd expect a day or so after a missed period."

That wasn't right. My hCG should have been way above that by now and producing a strong reading on that test. My hCG must only be around 20, barely able to get a reading on a 50 hCG test. At that moment I was gripped with another paralysing pain in my back and had to be wheeled out to the car in a wheelchair. What on earth was going on?

Year 3, Tuesday 24 July—
Hunstanton

It was time to hit the road again. Dad was feeling a little better although he still didn't feel like eating. My back was still having spasms and I was depleted of energy but if we didn't get a move on now, we'd miss catching up with my mum's sister, my Aunty May.

We had booked into a 'sea side chalet' which, in English terms, proved to be four cold walls with bunk beds, no shower and a single fan heater to warm the coldest of days. Clearly not the holiday we were expecting and with all of us suffering the flu, it wasn't going to be a pleasant experience. The Panadol I was taking for my back pain seemed to be taking the edge off of the uninviting environment. My Aunty May had joined us and was the only one who didn't have the lurgy—yet. She was a welcome burst of jovial energy in what has been a mundane few days.

It was our first night in Hunstanton and we were desperately trying to make the most of the situation. We headed across to the chalet dining area to grab a bite to eat and watch some free live entertainment. Braving the bone chilling winds, we found ourselves a table and Fez bought a round of drinks even though no-one really felt like drinking. There was a duo playing on the stage and the dance floor was full of senior citizens line-dancing to anything with a beat. We took a few happy snaps and had a good chuckle at the line-dancers' expense.

We returned to the chalet and checked on dad who had gone back to being incapacitated in bed. Mum put the kettle on as we all got ready for bed. I was desperate for the toilet, so I put on my thick woolly PJ's and made my way to the bathroom. The tiles were like icicles on my bare feet. I squatted carefully over the cracked toilet seat and peered inside the toilet bowl, only to see thick red blood running down the side of the toilet. The back spasms had, in fact, been my uterus contracting so violently that I had lost my baby down a cold, rusted pipe. I despised Hunstanton.

The countryside of Hunstanton still brings a chill to my spine. It was quite possibly the worst four days of my life.

Year 3, Wednesday 25 July—
Nothing

I can't remember anything about last night. My Aunty said she found me on the bathroom tiles clutching at bloodied toilet paper in a frantic state. She said I had called out for mum, but mum had gone to the car.

There wasn't any medical help close to Hunstanton so I was left to endure the physical and emotional fall-out of my miscarriage. My baby, gone. Our baby, gone. Each breath was like gasping for life. My sweet baby. I have to leave you here. Why me? I knew something was wrong. I knew my pregnancy hormone levels weren't as they should be but I never thought this would happen. I didn't think life could be so cruel after all we'd been through. We were on our holiday. We were trying to forget. We wanted this baby so much.

Year 3, Tuesday 31 July—
Breaking the news

As each new morning comes and goes, I relive the pain of losing our baby, of no longer feeling the excitement of waking up being pregnant, and the despair of having the infertility monkey back on my back. The pregnancy tests stare at me as a constant reminder of the hope that I had just a few days ago. The fact that this has happened on our well-earned holiday is even more devastating and cruel. What could we have done to deserve this?

After a few more days of travelling I plucked up the courage to text the few of my friends and family that have been told the good news. Only now, the news is brief and to the point:

"Hi guys. We jumped the gun. I miscarried a few days ago, lost the baby. Oh well, keep trying I guess . . . Deb x"

True to form, my text message managed to be devoid of the true gut wrenching despair I was feeling.

I was glad to be over on the other side of the world and able to take solace in the fact that I wouldn't have to face anyone. I missed a lot of good time with the family because I was simply not present and I regret that so much. But I may as well not be here at all. I'm sure my family have noticed how distant I am. I tried desperately to get some medical help to confirm my miscarriage and find out what went wrong but I am at a loss to find the kind of help and answers I need. The only help I received was through a healthcare hotline where the nurse listened to my story sympathetically over the telephone and assured me that miscarriage is a very common occurrence and that at six weeks there shouldn't be any need for medical intervention. It still didn't give me any answers as to WHY I lost my baby. I would continue to suffer in silence.

I'm relieved that the best part of our holiday is still to come. Tomorrow, Fez and I will set off alone to the romance of Italy, Croatia and our final destination, Santorini, leaving Hunstanton behind us.

Year 3, Wednesday 1 August—
Oceans of love

Here, in Santorini, I lay my baby to rest and cast my heart's sorrow and grief into the beautiful ocean that lies before me. Goodbye. And with that comes the thought: I can get pregnant naturally. If the Chinese herbs worked this month, what is to stop them from working next month? We are in the perfect location so we will keep trying.

Year 3, Monday 6 August—
Everything must come to an end

Today marks the final day of our European vacation. It is beautiful here. The kind of beauty that can make you cry involuntarily. We have made love every single day. We are simply not going to miss an opportunity and I'll be damned if I am coming home from our trip-of-a-lifetime still infertile. A tiny little light is beginning to shine at the end of the tunnel. It has been the best and worst times of my life, all in four weeks.

CHAPTER 11

Que sera sera

> "Que Sera Sera . . . Whatever will be, will
> be. The future's not ours to see. Que Sera
> Sera."—RAY EVANS

Year 3, Tuesday 21 August—
Back to the real world

We arrived back on Aussie soil, and it wasn't long before
I had my period and was back to square one. I made
another appointment with my Chinese doctor and told
her what happened. We then went about plotting another
course of disgusting, dirt-tasting herbs. She reassured me
that we would take 'strengthening' herbs this time once a
pregnancy is achieved—just to give my body some extra
reinforcement. She has dealt with a lot of women with
recurring miscarriages. During my consultation, she talked
about her work with some of the local universities and in

particular discussed a study on Chinese medicine run in conjunction with IVF.

During my appointment, a doctor's name came up in conversation that a lot of patients have been referred to. His name is Dr Mark Livingstone. I rang. The waiting list to get an appointment with him was long. We are already on a long waiting list with the clinic but, as coincidence would have it, Dr Livingstone had a cancellation and we managed to get an appointment scheduled for a few weeks time.

Year 3, Tuesday 11 September— *Dr Mark Livingstone*

When we eventually met with Dr Livingstone, I felt a huge weight lift off my shoulders. He was younger than I had imagined, with a thick Scottish accent. There was a sincerity and a credibility about him that made me believe him when he said I would fall pregnant. We discussed our previous history more thoroughly than I had ever done before. We discussed our prior failed attempts and showed him copies of all our lab reports. After careful consideration he laid out a plan of action for our first cycle. We would have to start from scratch with a fresh cycle, but this time the difference would be the advanced laboratory techniques. Genea leads the world in the use of day five blastocyst transfers. This means the embryo is in a more advanced stage of cell division. It's the final stage of development, before the embryo hatches out of the outer shell and is ready for implantation. That's the simplest way for me to explain it. If the embryo survives to day three, they will continue to support its development in the lab. If it makes it to day five we then would have a 50% chance of achieving a pregnancy from each embryo transfer. The other clinic transfers on day three after a 'not so advanced' culture. It is like a light has gone off inside my head. Why didn't I find out this information at the start? I am kicking myself.

We also discussed that if we still don't have a positive outcome after two more attempts, then we should consider having a laparoscopy. This involves keyhole surgery into the abdomen to check out the lining of the uterus to see if there is any scar tissue or endometriosis that is preventing successful implantation. I realise now that if we want to progress with treatment, then I will have to agree to having some kind of investigative surgery if IVF fails again. Other than that, we have to wait for the next menstrual cycle before we can start treatment to give my body a chance to get rid of any residual pregnancy hormones that are still present in my body. Then we would need to attend an orientation briefing at the clinic where we will collect the IVF drugs and information pack.

We left his office with the reassurance that there isn't any reason we shouldn't achieve success with IVF. It is just a matter of when. I am feeling excited to start on a new journey and feel pleased with myself for taking charge of the situation this time. I feel like we're on the right track and exactly where we should be. This time I am in charge of my fertility fate.

Year 3, Wednesday 19 September—
If I knew then, what I know now.

When I look back, I realise it's been a year now since we started on this IVF journey. I've learned so much since then and been through so much. I've encountered some fairly major hurdles that would make or break some people, but I'm still here. Still trying, still somehow believing that there is a chance for me.

It's time to start the whole process again with a renewed enthusiasm. With all this additional knowledge comes the realisation that it is possible that none of our eggs will make it to the day five blastocyst stage, leaving us with nothing to transfer at the end of the cycle. This isn't uncommon for women who have few eggs at retrieval. I can't imagine what it would be like to go through the gruelling IVF drug stimulation and have nothing to transfer at the end of it. Some specialists believe an embryo has a much better chance of developing further when transferred back into the uterus, the most natural of environments, as early as possible. The trouble with this however is that most embryos arrest in the day three to five stage. As I am finding out there is always a positive and negative to every facet of IVF.

My attitude towards this is if things haven't worked previously, why repeat them? I am open and willing to try the day five procedure.

The other major difference with this new clinic, apart from the advanced culture, is that the down regulation drug is given by injection rather than nasal spray. I am also put on the pill before commencing treatment. The extra injection a day is not pleasant but this is the approach Dr Livingstone has designed for me and is how it is done at Genea and I trust his plan of treatment. Genea's success rates speak for themselves. I will also be fully conscious and awake during egg retrieval, as the needle is guided into my ovaries under a simple local anaesthetic. I wonder why they put me under at the other clinic? I never questioned it. I thought it was all part of the procedure. Dr Livingstone explained that the option to have anaesthetic is a personal one that should be discussed with your doctor and that I can request it if I like but there isn't any real necessity for it. I think I'd rather be awake. It's a scary prospect—but no scarier than the thought of never waking from a general anaesthetic.

Year 3, Thursday 20 September—
I wonder . . .

We are approaching the end of the year and there are many social events to attend so I try to carry on with day-to-day life as much as possible, even drinking alcohol whenever the opportunity presents itself. I've had enough sacrifice. I am not going to spend another month punishing myself for having a mere glass or two of wine. It helps me relax and takes the edge off the harsh reality of knowing we're facing another Christmas without a family.

Work has stepped up another notch and bookings are coming in thick and fast for the corporate Christmas season. It's always a relief to know where the dollars are coming from. It will help us pay off the credit card and put aside some savings for next year. This time of the year usually flies by and I'd be lying if I said I couldn't be happier to see the end of this year.

In a few days it will be my 36th birthday. I haven't planned anything. It's just another birthday. I'm on the cusp of being at the 'older' end of the age spectrum for IVF. Fantastic. Today I took a walk to the shops and saw a heavily pregnant lady crossing the road at a pedestrian crossing. My mind wandered. What would life be like if we fast forwarded one year from now. Maybe I would be crossing that same street heavily pregnant. Maybe I would be pushing a stroller. I prayed with all my might that this was our last Christmas without a baby to hold. I decided not to put the Christmas tree up this year. Seemed pointless. Maybe next year.

I got home to find my period had started. Time to call the clinic.

Year 3, Tuesday 2 October—
Text book cycle

We have finished our first Genea cycle and in the next 24 hours I will have the trigger injection. This is the mother of all injections. As we have experienced previously, this has to be timed meticulously and given at the exact time of day the clinic specifies or else you throw your cycle into jeopardy. Mine just so happens to be scheduled right while I am on stage in the middle of my set at a corporate band gig in the beautiful Hunter Valley north of Sydney.

I have it all planned. Fez will travel with me to the gig as my driver and when the moment comes—9.15 pm to be precise—I will excuse myself from the stage by whispering something into my guitarist's ear and bolt for the disabled toilet to administer my egg releasing drug. How incredibly rock and roll of me, shooting up mid-way through my gig in the toilets!

Year 3, Wednesday 3 October—
Hunter Valley 9.15 pm

I had about two minutes to get the deed done. I ran offstage. Fez stood waiting in the toilet cubicle, needle poised. I lifted my top, pinched a layer of fat and waited for the jab. Done. Bolted back to stage and made it back in time to resume the third verse. Phew. The song was "Ain't Nobody . . . does it better". Poignant.

Year 3, Friday 5 October—
Two Short of Two Dozen

Exactly 36 hours after my trigger shot I was back in the familiar white walls of our new clinic, waiting for my Doctor to arrive. I was dressed in a hospital gown and sitting anxiously on a leather recliner. The only thing separating me from the ten or so other women waiting was a wrap-around hospital curtain. I pondered over my file.

Dr Livingstone was running half an hour late and by the time he arrived emotions were running high in the clinic. I strained to hear a conversation coming from a few curtain booths down. At first, it is just hushed whispers. I could detect Dr Livingstone's accent. The whispers soon turned into gut-wrenching sobs. It was hard to block out the drama.

The sobbing continued for what seemed like an eternity. I began to grow more and more nervous about our own prospects. We were still waiting for our egg retrieval but what if something went wrong? What if we had missed the ovulation period altogether? Sometimes it is possible for the eggs to be released sooner than the 36 hour trigger injection window.

That would be a whole month of treatment down the drain and a month is forever in the fertility cycle. I leaned back and closed my eyes. I felt for this poor woman and her partner. It was a devastating reality check that sometimes, no matter how far you took this IVF game and how many attempts you could emotionally endure, it just may not work.

My thoughts were interrupted by one of the clinic's nurses. As she entered our booth, Dr Livingstone followed and slid his back down the wall to sit on the floor, as if with a huge sigh of relief to be rid of the emotional situation he had just endured. I wanted to ask what was going on but thought I would be considered too nosey. Doctor Livingstone explained the all too familiar procedure.

Before making my way into the egg retrieval room, I had a joke with Dr Livingstone that my pet cocky was also harvesting eggs and, over the past few weeks, was now one short of laying a dozen. I told him that we were having a little competition and it was my aim to get 12 eggs so we could be on par. He indulged me and at the end of the procedure, poked his head back into the recovery room to tell me I had in fact beaten the cocky. I had produced 22 good-looking eggs! Whoa, 22 eggs. Two shy of TWO dozen. That was a heck of a lot of potential embryos. And so the journey towards fertilisation had begun—again.

Year 3, Saturday 6 October—
Fertilisation report

I am feeling confident about our chances. Being a numbers game, the greater the numbers, the better the odds. Exactly 24 hours after the harvest we were informed by our nurse that 18 eggs had fertilised and we would now have to wait to see how many made it to blastocyst. This is the scary part. It will be a long five-day wait.

Year 3, Wednesday 10 October—
Five days past egg collection

Out of 22 eggs, we got 7 viable blastocysts with each embryo having its own 50/50 chance of resulting in a pregnancy. This was great news. We couldn't have hoped for anything better. It made it even clearer to me the difference in day three and day five culture system.

The embryo transfer was all set for this afternoon and Dr Livingstone informed us that due to my age and the quality of the embryos, only one embryo should be transferred and the remaining could, if desired, be frozen for future IVF attempts. IVF in Australia has certain standards to ensure that multiple pregnancies are avoided wherever possible. Genea strongly support single embryo transfers and as much as I would leap at the opportunity to increase my chances by having multiple embryos transferred, it was explained that this was the procedure that would serve us best. Usually if a woman is 35 and under, one single embryo is placed back into the uterus as the odds of achieving a successful pregnancy are still quite considerable. Over the age of 36, the odds decrease and sometimes a woman could have more than one embryo transferred in an attempt to increase conception success, but this is done very rarely. I was happy with all that. I have my hopes pinned on that number one embryo.

"Good news," said the scientist. "This one is continuing to progress and is hatching as we speak."

She explained how one half of the figure eight goes on to become the placenta once it attaches itself in the uterus. The other half would potentially become the egg sac. It sounded complicated but I was very pleased with our A grade embryo and was growing more and more confident by the minute. The procedure was over in the blink of an eye. Dr Livingstone liked to give a vaginal probe ultrasound to check that the embryo has entered the uterus. So there, right before our eyes, on the monitor is a tiny little white speck that resembles nothing more than an air bubble and a lifetime of hope.

Year 3, Sunday 14 October—
Patience is a virtue

Again, the two week wait is murderous. You can never 'just relax' or not think about it. As the day draws closer, the temptation to pee on a stick is like the unopened box of chocolates tempting you from the couch. I know better. If it's negative, I'll be devastated. If it's positive, I'll obsess over its validity and whether that damn line is telling me the truth or not.

It has been four days since embryo transfer and I have a realisation that I am actually nine days past ovulation (or when my eggs were harvested) which means a home pregnancy test could detect a pregnancy if it was sensitive enough. It is like a bolt of lightning has hit me in the head. Here I am expecting to wait out the full 14 days after egg collection, when I could technically test from today given the fact that our embryo was transferred at five days past ovulation. I am going to wait until tomorrow morning's pee.

Year 3, Monday 15 October—
Pessimist

I waited until the first sign of daylight to take the dreaded test. The test line came up almost immediately followed by a second positive indicator line. The trigger shot couldn't still be in my system this late, so here I was, once again, 'pregnant'. Why wasn't I more excited?

I paused for a long moment on the toilet seat and recalled the various occasions this past year where I had been in this exact same situation and, for some reason, this time round, my reaction was just not quite what I'd hoped it would be. With any initial excitement comes the dreaded anxiety and this time it's popped up first, stealing my moment, filling me with fear again. I am all too familiar with what lies ahead of me and what could go wrong.

Year 3, Wednesday 17 October—
Secret power

I've been carrying around my little secret for over a day now. I've held back on blurting out the news of my positive pregnancy test as if playing a game with the test itself. I don't have to believe that stick. It's been nothing but an object of misery to me and I would not let it get my hopes up again, only to destroy me later. I haven't told a soul, not even Fez or mum yet. After all, how many times have they had this same conversation with me. It was tainted.

"Yes, we're pregnant . . . oops, hold on a minute . . . no we're not. Sorry guys! I'm wrong again."

It is almost a joke. My blood pregnancy test is on Friday. Just the rest of today and one whole day tomorrow to wait. The hours are passing slowly. I keep checking my underwear for any sign of a period. Dry. Sore boobs—no. Emotional—always. Optimistic?—better leave that blank. I decided to tell Fez. I chose my words carefully and, with the announcement, received a reserved hug and words of congratulations. It just isn't the same. I guess it never will be.

Year 3, Friday 19 October—
The reveal

As the official blood pregnancy test grew closer, I became increasingly tempted to pee on another stick. Today, the morning of my appointment at the clinic, I did so. My stick still showed a positive result but when I really analysed it, the line was fractionally lighter than it was before. I refused to play mind games with myself anymore and threw both sticks away. My eyes could be playing tricks on me. There was no point. I would wait for the official result this afternoon.

Midday rolled around and the clinic was yet to call with my results once again. History repeating itself. They said they would ring around midday. It was 2.00 pm and I was beside myself. Fez and I were both pacing our tiny one bedroom apartment. I called them, left a message, called them back. Eventually my mobile rang. I recognised the clinic's number on my caller ID immediately. I took a deep breath and announced to Fez that this was it. My head was spinning.

"Mrs Krizak? This is Sydney IVF. We have the results of your blood test this morning. Are you somewhere where we can talk?"

"Yes, yes," hurrying her along.

"Well, Mrs Krizak . . . Unfortunately the result of your test is a non-viable pregnancy."

"Non-viable? What exactly does that mean?"

She didn't say "negative", she said "non-viable".

"I'm so sorry Mrs Krizak. It just means that the embryo did attach and started to secrete hCG but it didn't develop for long enough to be considered viable. We like the hCG levels to be somewhere around 50-100 at this stage and your reading was just 7. It's what we call a biochemical pregnancy".

"So it's not a miscarriage?"

"No, it's way too early in the development to be considered a miscarriage. You won't need any treatment for it. You'll just get a slightly heavier bleed in the next few days and it may be a little uncomfortable."

I didn't hear any more but I already knew that the feeling I was feeling was a lot more than 'a little uncomfortable'. My heart was broken. Fez was there to carry me as I put down the phone. I didn't need to even explain to him what had happened. I sobbed and sobbed in his arms. When would this ever end? This was the cruelest blow.

Year 3, Saturday 20 October— Time for Plan B

I want to rid myself of this past year's expectation on myself to get pregnant. Dealing with failure is one thing, but knowing that despite all my best efforts, some things just will not go to plan makes the magnitude of the frustration so much bigger. Should we keep on going and relive this nightmare? Or should we accept our fate, take some time to grieve and start planning for our future in a different way? I think by this stage we had both realised that we would not have children of our own. And even though the thought and desire was heavy in our hearts, the burden of failed attempt after failed attempt was much more than we were prepared to put ourselves through.

Dr Livingstone made a caring follow-up call to see how I was getting on and to outline a future plan of action. I felt like I had become that desperate woman we heard in the clinic just a few weeks ago. I told Dr Livingstone that we didn't have any plans to continue and that we were going to take some time out to think through our options. He must have heard this a million times before.

"Look Deb," he said matter of factly. "You have six frozen embryos, just give the clinic a call when you want to go ahead with an FET. You can start straight away if you like. You don't even need to make an appointment to come and see me. It's very straight forward and you've got six good blastocysts there. I'm sorry this one didn't work out for you."

Year 3, Monday 22 October—
What makes a good parent?

The reality has already sunk in. It's only been two days but my mind is going 24/7. I have thought about the prospect of adoption and thrown myself into finding out as much about the process as possible. I contacted Department of Community Services (DOCS) and asked how we could go about becoming eligible adoptive parents. All I needed to know about the initial stages of adopting a child from overseas was sent to me by email. If we were accepted initially, we would have to attend a preliminary adoption seminar, followed by an intensive weekend course as well as extensive psychological testing. All of this didn't sound too appealing to Fez but, in my desperation, he agreed to let me fill out the application and we would go from there. I got started immediately. I was a woman on a mission.

I sat at my computer and went through the application process. It was confronting. Questions such as "why would you make good parents?" and "have you undergone fertility treatment in the past?" They all bring up those familiar feelings of failure and despair. How would I justify why we would make great parents after having gone through a year of feeding myself hormones and enduring every kind of invasive procedure, in the hope of producing a child of our own? This would let them know how much I really wanted a child to love but what does it say about me as a parent? To top it all off, there was the application fee that we have to pay just to get someone to read 'why we would make great parents'. What were we getting ourselves into? I mulled over my answers and pressed 'send'. Initial application sent. Where did today go?

Year 3, Tuesday 23 October—
No time to waste

I received a phone call from DOCS saying we had been selected to attend the preliminary adoption course this weekend if we were available. It took me a few minutes to register who I was talking to. I expected to wait months to hear back from them. I only sent the application forms off yesterday! Turns out, they had two places available this Sunday for the adoption seminar and were offering this vacancy to us first. I was impressed with how quickly things were moving. It had all gone quite smoothly so far and I welcomed the change. Perhaps this was the path we were meant to end up on all along. I was beginning to feel liberated again. We were a happily married couple, married almost nine years in fact, owned several properties and were financially secure. What better candidates could they possibly find? It all seemed pretty straight forward to me. I paid with my credit card over the phone to secure our attendance at the seminar. I didn't think twice about the $200 price tag and broke the news to Fez that his usual Sunday, reserved for football, would now be spent watching videos of orphaned children and matching us up with a child to bring home.

Year 3, Sunday 28 October—
Bubble bursts . . .

Life has taken a 360 degree turn. I am now completely obsessed with the romance of adoption. The celebrities all do it. I couldn't sleep last night contemplating which country we would pursue for adoption. I couldn't wait to find out each and every detail.

It was the first of the preliminary adoption workshops. Fez was sceptical. I walked in and felt immediately comforted by being in a room with others who have had fertility problems. It was nice to be away from the fertile world that surrounds me every day and to chat to other couples about their own journeys.

They screened a video featuring an adopted woman venturing back to her birth country to meet her biological family. She had been adopted out at two years of age and did not have any memory of her birth parents. Her search and quest to find them hit me hard. It was as if the true essence of her soul could not rest until she found these people. Even though she came from a loving American family who had supported her the whole way through, she was still driven to find her natural parents. It is a deep, basic genetic need that should never be denied for an adopted child or adult. This got me thinking. As an adoptive parent, could I live with this child's overwhelming desire to one day find their own biological family? This was really confronting. Could I go through hell and back to adopt a child, give them all the love and support in the world, foregoing many of my own needs along the way, only to find that quite possibly, in the end, it may never be enough. Could I cope with the reality that the urge to find one's genetic history and belonging is far more powerful than my love could ever be?

The day concluded, and we were given a folder filled with long-winded application forms and case studies of other families to read through. Now the race would begin to get the application in as soon as possible. It would be no easy feat and would take months of character references, medical records and constant psych evaluation. I turned to face Fez, only to notice he was no longer sitting beside me. I couldn't see him anywhere in the room. After a few minutes, I excused myself and made my way out to the foyer where he was waiting for me.

"Good," he said. "Then you agree, adoption's not for us. I couldn't go through all that after what we've been through already."

I nodded in half-hearted submission but realised he was right. We both had to let the pain go and deal with our loss of not being able to become parents of our own genetic offspring first before we could digest the magnitude of the adoption process. It is a brave realisation but necessary for us to move forward. I had thrown us into another pit of disappointment without giving any validation to the feelings we were already dealing with. It was easier to mask those feelings than deal with them head on. I guess it was now or never.

I don't want to be taken the wrong way here, adoption works wonderfully for many families, but it's so important to be at peace about the decision. We aren't there yet. Adoptive parents have to be willing to accept the long, uncertain road towards bringing that child into their world, and that could take more strength than I think I could ever muster.

Year 3, Monday 29 October— *Grey skies are gonna clear up . . . Put on a happy face*

What now? Another year has come and almost gone. The year of the IVF! We'd started in January and it was now the end of October and I am already 36.

It was a friend's 40th tonight, but we didn't feel much like celebrating, so we opted for a quiet night at home and talked of a better year ahead. Fez and I fantasised about all the wonderful things we could do together in the years to come. Holidays, buy more properties and enjoy the simple life of a couple without commitments. Yes, we wouldn't be like everyone else but we'd find a way to fit in. And when it all got too much we could hop on a plane and go to some exotic destination and sip cocktails while they were all up every three hours with desperate, crying babies. Simple. We could even end up the envy of all our friends.

It was hard to not look back on the year and be overwhelmed by feelings of failure. The constant, nagging sadness is like a rotating lead weight in the pit of my stomach. It never goes away. It just keeps turning and turning, slowly grinding away and reminding me. It keeps me awake at night and overrides any brief moments of happiness that life throws at us. From the outside looking in, we are a normal, happy couple able to enjoy social events and time spent together, but in reality is what people don't see—the void that we are left with, behind closed doors and in the dark of night. Yes, I can put on a smile and a face in my professional life. That's part of my job. I guess many couples don't last the threat of infertility but somehow we have managed to hold on for dear life and turn to each other when we have needed it the most. In that respect, we are blessed. Things could have turned out completely differently.

Year 3, Wednesday 31 October—
Wedding proposal

We were out to dinner with our dear friends Mel and Mario who have been trying to set a date for their wedding but hadn't, we thought, decided where. Sometime before main course and after a second bottle of wine, they announced they would be eloping to Las Vegas to get married. They have plans to visit the strip and get married at the Little White Wedding Chapel, by none other than the man himself, Elvis. They invited us to come along, which sounded fun. Then they dropped the bombshell. The wedding is next weekend! Three empty bottles of wine later and memories fresh from our European vacation only three months earlier, we shook hands and agreed to be witnesses at their marriage. It felt strangely liberating deciding to do something so random right there and then and a spark of excitement began to grow from that miserable pit of sadness within me. We were going to Vegas baby and I couldn't wait! What a wonderful belated birthday surprise to myself. That's how I'd justify incurring more credit card debt—a birthday treat. I didn't get any resistance from Fez. It might just be the best birthday after all! This certainly has been the most stressful and carefree year rolled into one. Stressful for the obvious reasons, carefree when it came to finances.

Year 3, Friday 9 November— ## *Vegas baby!*

The day after the dinner party we purchased flights and arranged accommodation in Vegas, which our friends were kind enough to pay for. Just under a week later we boarded the flight, our heads in a spin and giggling like kids on a school excursion. We arrived in Los Angeles severely sleep deprived and headed for our friends house in the Hollywood Hills for a few days before setting off to Vegas. There wasn't a thing to do but shop, sample the nightlife and wrangle our way into restaurants that were usually reserved for the rich and famous. We were having the time of our lives. It was just what the Chinese doctor would have ordered.

Year 3, Wednesday 14 November—
Jet Lag

Back home. We arrived late in the evening after an initial delay from Los Angeles. The wedding was fun, heartfelt and silly with 'Elvis' delivering more than just 'one for the money' on numerous occasions throughout the twenty minute service. We all laughed a lot at the craziness of the situation but were also completely blown away by the love that our two friends shared.

If ever there had ever been a perfect moment in time to conceive, this would have been it. I have never been happier, more relaxed or open minded. It just goes to show that not everyone's right when they tell couples who are trying for a baby to 'take a holiday, forget about it and it'll happen'. We'd been waiting a very long time if there was any truth in that statement.

This new frame of mind made me think about our remaining six embryos and whether we could use some of this renewed energy to give it one more bash before the year was out. Financially, it made sense as we were still covered by the Medicare threshold rebate until the new year kicked in. What the heck. They were just sitting there anyway and I had all but given up hope. I called the clinic and explained to the nurse where I was in my cycle—roughly around day 12. Could be cutting it fine. Hopefully I hadn't ovulated yet and we could squeeze a transfer in this month. Booked in for a blood test tomorrow morning and we'd take it from there. Why not give it one last bash? If not for us, then for Elvis. In celebration of our fabulous trip to Vegas.

Year 3, Friday 16 November—
Not one but two

IVF # 4. FET. Two embryos are thawed, both survived. One with 20% loss of cells and graded B and C grade respectively. Like the Vegas trip, this FET was spontaneous and exciting. My hormones were spot on and I didn't have any time to ponder the IVF fallout game.

The process was exactly the same as our previous IVF, except we had already produced the embryos and they only had to survive the hurdle of being 'defrosted'.

Dr Livingstone approached me to discuss the option of transferring 2 embryos back into the uterus as I had had several previous unsuccessful cycles. Technically, I am a little young to be transferring two well-developed embryos, but his thinking was nothing has worked in the past, so we would increase our chances of success. Dr Livingstone specialises in the prevention of multiple pregnancy which often puts IVF patients in the high risk category if they fall pregnant with twins or more. His mission is to achieve a singleton pregnancy with the best possible live birth rate, keeping potential risk factors to a minimum. You hear about multiple embryo implantation a lot overseas, where women fall pregnant with an unheard of amount of babies, only to risk severe pre-term delivery and the life of themselves and their children. In Australia we are very conservative with embryo transfers to prevent the possibility of multiple pregnancy. It's too risky all round and is not something that clinics will automatically proceed with. For Fez and I, the fact that we had unexplained infertility, produced abundant embryos and responded well to the meds, meant that it was simply a numbers game and placing two embryos back into the uterus seemed to be a sensible solution to beating these odds.

I didn't spare a thought about having two embryos put back in. I got to see both dancing figure eights on the clinic's widescreens and was fascinated to discover that it was general practice at Genea for all frozen embryos to undergo assisted hatching. This is where a tiny hole is made in the outer layer of the embryo shell to encourage it to break out and attach to the uterine lining. The embryologist explained that sometimes, with age and the freezing process, the zona (or egg shell) becomes tougher than normal and can make it harder for the egg itself to hatch. I was thrilled to know we were pulling out all the stops and trying something we had never done before. I was fascinated.

Year 3, Sunday 25 November—
End of the year. End of the road. Again.

This time the dreaded two week wait has just flown by and I have had a completely different attitude towards it.

I don't believe for a minute that the FET has worked. As a result I am eating and drinking my way merrily through the lead up to the silly season without sparing a thought for my B and C grade hatching blastocysts floating around in my endometrium. There are no symptoms to suggest I am pregnant. No sore boobs, nausea or "hunches". It is business as usual.

Just before bed tonight I found one of my remaining pregnancy tests and decided to use it there and then. After all, the definitive result will be revealed tomorrow. No more waiting. I placed the home pregnancy test in my urine stream and waited the usual few minutes for it to decide my fate. As predicted, there was only one pink line and a very strong negative jumping out to wish me goodnight. I placed the stick on the bathroom basin and put myself to bed, not uttering a word to Fez.

CHAPTER 12

Don't count your chickens . . .

**"You can leave your own mark behind by
making a difference in this world, maybe not
genetically but spiritually and emotionally."**

Year 3, Monday 26 November—
Rumbling vibration

I woke, got dressed, went in for the blood test and took
myself off to a casting for a TV show and put my mobile
phone on silent. The casting was a welcome diversion but
I was mostly excited about mum arriving in a few hours
time. Fez had gone to the airport to pick her up while I was
out. Before he left, I told Fez about last night's negative
pregnancy test, mostly to break the anguish of receiving
the "not pregnant" sympathy call from the clinic. I couldn't
tell if he was upset at the news or angry at me for breaking
the rules again and taking the test. When I got home mum

was there and we sat down, had a glass of wine and a cuddle on the couch.

Mid afternoon rolled around and mum and I decided to go out for a bit of retail therapy. I told her about this last FET attempt but proceeded to tell her that it was unsuccessful. I hadn't even told her I went for a blood test that morning. It wasn't of any importance anymore. We had a lovely afternoon shopping and decided to stop for a coffee and a bite to eat. Just then I felt my phone vibrating in my bag as it sat on my lap. I eventually found the phone and realised I had left it on silent the whole day. I have seven missed calls. They are all from the same number. I excused myself to retrieve my voicemail messages in a quieter area. Suddenly I was in a daze of anticipation. I made my way to the closest fire escape corridor and dialled my voicemail.

The first message is from Dr Livingstone. A message of congratulations. The second is from a very excited nurse dying to tell me that she had some VERY GOOD NEWS and that I should call immediately as it may make my weekend a lot more exciting. From then on, it is repeated return calls from both Dr Livingstone and the nurses. All of them are bursting to tell me the good news. Finally after a year of waiting for the damn phone to ring, I left it on silent and missed the very call I'd been dreaming about for so long. My God. I was unable to hold the phone anymore as my knees are giving way.

Somewhere in a maze of confusion I managed to call the nurses and sat speechless as they congratulated me with the news that I had a very positive blood pregnancy result with an hCG reading of almost twice of what could be expected at this early pregnancy stage.

"So you had two embryos put back in" one of the nurses remarks. "Yes. Why? Do you think it could be twins?" "Well it's way too early to tell but it's a very strong hormone level. You'll find out soon enough at your seven week ultrasound. Good luck and continue to take your vaginal pessaries for the next five weeks until we see you next". I hung up the phone. I had a call waiting. It was Dr Livingstone.

"Congratulations Debora. I'm taking it you've heard the good news?" "Yes. I can't believe it Mark. I'm in shock. I'm sitting in a fire escape and I don't know what to do next".

"Well, take it easy and we'll see you in three weeks for your next ultrasound. It's a very solid pregnancy result so you should be happy." "Could it be twins?" "I'd say it's unlikely. Twins usually have a much higher hCG reading from my experience."

I ended the call expressing my shocked gratitude. I suddenly realised that I've left mum waiting at the café for a bit over 30 minutes. But I couldn't go back to her until I had spoken to Fez. I dialled his mobile and Fez answered almost immediately. I blurted out all the news at the speed of light and reassured him that I had been told this was a strong pregnancy result this time. He sounded as shocked as I was but there was a relief in his voice and a calmness I had not heard before.

"But you said this morning you took a test and it was negative."

"Yes I know," I said. "I don't understand that either. They said my hormone levels were quite high. I don't know why it didn't show up on the home pregnancy test." Finally I was convinced that those bloody things didn't actually work after all. Now I had proof. I made my way back to mum. She had gathered all our bags together and was just about to come looking for me. I explained that I had been on an important call to my agent and that I might need to dash off again if the phone rang. Mum completely bought my story and we set off to look for a Christmas present for my nephew Felix who was now 18 months old. I had no idea if this was the right time to tell mum or not but it was only a matter of time before she'd tune into my nervous energy. I decided to take her into a little clothing shop for kids. Staring out at me from the shop window was the opportunity I was looking for. I picked up a tiny little Tee Shirt with a slogan on it that said "I LOVE GRANDMA". "What do you think about this mum?" "Oh. That's way too small for Felix. That's for a newborn." "Yes. So . . . What do you think?" "Oh you mean for Jemma?" Jemma is mum's tiny Maltese terrier. I was beginning to think she'd never get the hint. "Mum. No. What do you think about this GRANDMA?" Mum did a double take and finally caught my train of thought.

"Yes mum . . ." I was crying by now, "You are going to be a Grandma. I'm pregnant. Found out just now". Mum and I embraced for what seemed like an eternity. We put on quite a show in that little clothing shop at Westfield Shopping Centre.

Year 3, Friday 30 November—
Cone of Silence

Concealing something from the world that you've wanted for so many years is an almost impossible feat. Firstly, everyone notices when you're not drinking. That was the biggest giveaway for me. Secondly, prior to now I was always being asked how the treatment was going by some of my closest friends. Quite frankly, I haven't even made it to five weeks yet, let alone the recommended 12. I know what can go wrong and that the rug could still be pulled out from under me at any moment, so I would hate to make that same mistake again. Nevertheless, I whispered to my two closest friends that we were five weeks along, mainly so I had an alibi at all the Christmas social events as well as someone to discreetly fill my wine glass with lime and soda, which can look suspiciously like a crisp glass of sauvignon blanc in the right light.

We plan to go home to Adelaide to spend Christmas with our families. By then I will be roughly eight weeks pregnant. We have decided we will tell all the family then. That's if mum can contain her excitement and keep it quiet long enough! In the meantime, we still have to get through the seven week ultrasound to establish if we have a heartbeat and a viable pregnancy. In so many cases, you hear of women going for their first ultrasound and nothing but a sack is remaining in the uterus. The heartbeat just stops for no apparent reason and there aren't any physical signs to suggest that the pregnancy has ceased.

Year 3, Monday 17 December—
Pregnant until proven otherwise

Time for our appointment for the seven week scan. I was expecting the worst. To heighten my insecurities, I don't have a single one of the pregnancy symptoms—enlarged breasts, nausea, and heightened sense of smell? It is making me wonder if there is actually anything going on in there.

We were guided into the ultrasound room and they ask all the usual questions.

"What is your name? How many embryos did you have put back? Was it a natural pregnancy? I thought that was a fairly obvious answer.

The sonographer smothered my abdomen with a cold jelly-like substance and asked me to lie back and get comfortable. My neck strained forward so I could see the TV monitor in front of me. I had no idea what I was looking for. To me it was just a big grey mass of white specks. Fez sat beside me on a little plastic chair holding my hand. I felt like the blood had been drained from my limbs and I could feel my icy cold hands against his.

The sonographer was busy clicking and recording data on her screen. The silence was killing me. Suddenly she stops.

"Ok, there are two!" she exclaimed in a thick joyous, Asian accent.

Suddenly I could see what looked like two sacs side by side with a little flickering light in the middle of each sac.

"There are two healthy heartbeats. Congratulations, it's twins."

The tears streamed silently down my face in a sea of pride. From nothing to two. This was it. This was our path. We were never meant to have one baby. We were meant to have twins. There were so many signs along the way. My mind flashed back to the holiday house where we had met that annoying couple with the spa, pestering us to look at endless photos of her twin grandchildren. Then there was the lady in the maternity ward at Ashford hospital, the one that I found myself drawn to when visiting baby Chelsea, who had just given birth to pre-term twins. They were all signs, but I had failed to recognise any of them. I was so caught up in the midst of my own pain and suffering.

Fez passed out in the chair beside me. Lost in my own thoughts I failed to notice when that happened. Apparently the word "twins" tipped him over the edge—literally.

Fez came to and we left the clinic. I called mum to tell her the news. She was waiting with baited breath for my call. I barely dialled the number before she picked up.

"Mum, we got a heartbeat but guess what?"

Mum is silent.

"We got two heartbeats. It's twins," I screamed.

It was then that I realised mum had me on speaker phone and dad was listening as well.

It's hard to gauge someone's emotion over the phone but I knew what this moment meant to both of them.

"Well you never did do anything in halves my darling. You always surpass every obstacle and achieve more than you could ever imagine. I prayed to God for you. Every single night."

She was right. God, it has been a battle and I've been through the thick and thin of it all. But I'm not used to giving up. Mum's words made me feel proud.

Back to my miracle . . .

Not one, but two tiny lives were growing inside of me. Could we be any luckier?

When we arrived at our apartment I searched out that home pregnancy test stick and found a strong red line in the results window. That little bloody stick tricked me. By some stroke of fate, the line hadn't come up the night before but it was certainly making its presence felt now.

Year 3, Friday 21 December—
Two little beans

Each day passes in a daze. I am existing in some surreal kind of world. Every morning I have to remind myself that I am not dreaming. For the first few minutes of every day I wake in a panic thinking it has all been some kind of strange dream. It is difficult to grasp. It is finally, really happening.

As a precaution and as a way to constantly monitor my growing beans, I have opted for an additional support service at the clinic—Miscarriage Management Program. This entitled me to regular blood tests and scans to check the development of the babies is on track. Having to wait for the 12 week ultrasound would kill me. Since finding out I was pregnant, I've had blood taken weekly, and every afternoon the nurses call me to let me know that my hCG levels are climbing at the expected rate. This is a huge relief. Every day I feel one step closer to our dream. The extra management cost is a bit more but it is worth it for peace of mind. All is progressing to plan.

Today, Dr Livingstone called me. He explained that as I am carrying twins, I am now considered to be a high risk pregnancy, and any number of factors could make the pregnancy trickier.

Before this phone call, I hadn't given any of these risks a second thought. But now there are things like twin-to-twin transfusion syndrome, premature delivery, incompetent cervix, risk of losing one twin, breech delivery and any number of other complications which can occur with multiple pregnancies. Suddenly there is a whole new list of factors to worry about, just when I thought I could finally sit back and enjoy this wonderful triumph of being pregnant.

I asked Dr Livingstone what the key to success was this time round. I mean, nothing had worked previously and suddenly, bang, we get pregnant with twins. Dr Livingstone said that it was simply the right timing. He likened it to lotto. Our numbers had finally come up and, in our case, they'd come up twice. I wonder if it was the herbs which I continued to take up until seven weeks. Maybe it was the assisted hatching or maybe just maybe, it was the low dose aspirin I had been sneakily taking in an attempt to replicate other women's successful IVF pregnancy rates overseas that I had read about online. It seems to be quite often prescribed for a particular blood disorder but on many occasions I had read that it was a normal inclusion for some clinics' treatments.

I mentioned both the Chinese herbs and the aspirin to my clinic nurse, she advised me to stop taking them immediately. According to her, these drugs could cause a miscarriage in themselves. I stop taking both immediately.

Year 3, Monday 24 December— *Christmas*

We're flying from Sydney to Adelaide to spend Christmas with our families for a week. It's a relief to finally be pregnant at Christmas. I'm eight weeks pregnant today and still not out of the danger zone, but I can't pass up this opportunity to tell the family. After all, we didn't know when we would be seeing them again in the flesh. We told our extended families the news and my favourite part was waiting for the initial excitement to die down before blurting out that it was twins. It's like the unexpected double layer of chocolate you find when biting into an ice cream cone. Sweet. Everyone was elated. There was so much to celebrate.

With the announcement comes the insecurity. All the memories of Hunstanton come flooding back. I try to stop my heart from racing by breathing deeply. I don't want anything to unsettle my growing embryos. I excuse myself and make my way to the bathroom to check that I'm OK. I am. No blood this time. Breathe. I do this every half an hour for the rest of the day.

Year 4, Monday 7 January—
Ten weeks

We arrived back in Sydney and today it was our ten week ultrasound. I was very anxious. Thankfully, we could see the hearts beating and the foetuses had grown considerably in just a few weeks. Each scan is emotional, so I came armed with tissues. It is still so unbelievable. This time we were given our first little ultrasound picture. I put it up on the fridge with our little beans clearly marked Twin A and Twin B. It is funny hearing them referred to as Twin A and B. It has something to do with their positioning in my uterus.

Everything is looking great and I can't wait for the next two weeks to pass, so I can finally share this wonderful news with the world and get the anxiety monkey off my back.

In the post a letter arrived from DOCS advising Fez and I that we had been accepted as one of only a few couples selected each year to be eligible for local adoption and can now adopt a child from within Australia. I marvelled at the irony of the situation.

Year 4, Tuesday 15 January—
The business of being pregnant

We have been organising hospitals, doctors and health insurance. I had no idea there was so much to plan. I decided to call a friend and ask her for advice on where to start. Of course, this meant I had to spill the beans—but for planning's sake, I could afford to tell one person. I decided to book into North Shore Private Hospital and eventually found myself an obstetrician by the name of Dr Michael Van Der Griend. He was a fairly casual guy who had a bit of experience with twin pregnancies and luckily he was able to take me on as a new patient.

Our 40 week due date is around 2 August but Michael assured me that full term for a multiple pregnancy is generally around 37 weeks. Most likely I would need a Caesarian delivery because it is safer with twins. I hadn't given much thought to the birthing process. My only concern was to minimise the risk to the babies and get them out as quickly and safely as possible. We agreed on a C-section and the date would be set later on in the pregnancy. My sole goal is to keep these babies inside me for as long as physically possible.

Year 4, Monday 21 January—
12 Weeks

We've made it to 12 weeks. Our ultrasound today was perfect and the babies are growing well. I was so relieved. Finally the moment has come and we can tell the world about our fantastic news. I know so many people will be happy for us. I have already written a heart-felt email with our grand announcement and saved it in our drafts folder weeks ago. Now I just have to hit send and our news will be off into cyberspace!

I couldn't sleep so I decided to get up and send the email so that it would be the first mail our friends got in their inbox when they turned on their computers in the morning. The moment I hit send felt like it had been a thousand years coming. I sat at the computer for a moment just to process the magnitude of what I had just announced. It felt like closure. Suddenly it dawned on me that it was 1.00 am in the morning, so with that done, I set off for bed, eagerly anticipating the flood of replies tomorrow.

I must have been dreaming when I felt a nagging need to wake up. An all too familiar feeling is warm against my skin. It is still pitch black dark, so I dragged myself out of bed to go to the toilet. In just two hours time, friends from all over the world would be reading about our good news. I looked down at my thighs. The presence of bright red blood struck me like a blow to the head. It is like waking up really fast from an intense dream. I felt myself being whooshed up into a tunnel. I thought I was about to lose consciousness right then but Fez had followed me into the bathroom. My brain was unable to cope with the information I was being fed. I am 12 weeks pregnant. I have just seen both strong heartbeats. I was haemorrhaging.

Fez drove me to the hospital. I tried to keep my legs elevated in an attempt to slow the bleeding. I got flashbacks of my mum telling me to do that in Hunstanton when she came back from the car. God, I have just told the world our news. How could life be so cruel? Not now, please don't let me lose them now. I've made it to 12 weeks.

It was 3.45 am in the morning. We went straight to emergency and were seen immediately because I was bleeding so heavily. I was put on a stretcher and the night nurse tried in vain to find a vein in my arm. In the process of trying to locate a vein to put a drip into my arm, the needle slipped and blood came gushing out in violent squirts. The white sheets of the hospital stretcher were now barely recognisable.

I had to wait half an hour before a young doctor assessed me. He had a shocking bedside manner. In a matter of moments he explained to me that the most likely cause of the bleeding is that I was miscarrying. I explained to him through desperate sobs, that we had only just seen both heart beats hours before and how could it be possible that we have lost them so soon after that? His reply deafened me:

"It is quite common. Often there is something wrong with the pregnancy and it just takes a bit longer for the foetus to come away."

I clutched at my tummy and screamed at him. I didn't know what else to do. I desperately hoped this was some kind of terrible nightmare that I would wake from soon. Please God, don't take my babies. They're mine now. I've had them for three whole months. Every inch of me depends on them. Every moment of my existence is lived for them. Please no.

I must have scared the young doctor away. Lucky, because I wanted to rip his head off for saying my babies have died. Moments later, an authoritative lady from another department comes in to see me. She must have heard about all the commotion. She took my hand and explained calmly that in 90% of cases, bleeding is not in fact due to miscarriage. She is speaking from experience. I don't know if it is her intention to just calm me down but I believed her. I will cling to any hope. She gave me a sanitary napkin to place between my legs to catch the blood and advised us to have another ultrasound to see what is going on. The only catch was, I would have to wait another three hours before a sonographer was able to see me.

6.00 am finally rolls around, the bleeding had slowed and I was transferred to the X-ray department. By this time I was shaking with fear. Fez held on to me so tightly it was almost as if he was there in the bed beside me. With my eyes firmly shut, the ultrasound commenced. I was too frightened to look up at the monitor for fear of realising my worst dreams. The monitor was a lot smaller than the one we are used to at the clinic. And there they are. Two beating hearts. And no indication of what is causing the blood loss.

Year 4, Thursday 7 February—
Sub-Chorionic Haematoma

The bleeding has continued for two weeks now. I managed to see my OB and he sent me off for more detailed ultrasounds. In the meantime, I cannot live with the constant doubt over whether my babies have survived another day, so I hired a foetal Doppler which enables me to hear both heartbeats at any time of the day or night. I can't speak highly enough of this invention. It saved me from many an anxious moment, particularly as I was not at the stage where I could really feel any movement yet. I hired the Doppler for three months and planned to listen to those heartbeats at every possible opportunity.

Eventually, I was diagnosed as having a Sub-Chorionic Haematoma. In layman's terms, this means bleeding from within the uterus that is independent of the babies' environment, with the blood travelling down between the twin membrane which separates both sacs and gathers at the top of the cervix. I was told that in the course of a week or two, the bleeding should subside.

Year 4, Friday 15 February—
15 Weeks

I'm still bleeding. Just when I think it's stopped, I pass more clots and heavy bright red blood. It is a rollercoaster ride and one that leaves me fearing constantly for my babies. Instead of enjoying the experience of finally being pregnant, I am now living in fear of losing them. It is such an awful position to be in. I read that a mother's stress can have a negative effect on a baby while inside the womb. This creates even more stress.

Year 4, Monday 18 February—
16 Weeks

I am still having regular weekly monitoring. At my appointment with Dr Van der Griend I mentioned that the bleeding is persisting. He said that it is not normal to be bleeding this much at 16 weeks—and that this is a serious threat to the continuation of the pregnancy. He advised me to take it as easy as possible and if all continued to go well, to come back for my 18 week scan in two weeks time. There is something about the way he says "the 18 week scan" that makes me think he does not believe I will be walking through these doors again.

I am riddled with fear and have just about lost all hope. I want this damn bleeding to stop, to prove him wrong and to show others that sometimes bleeding does occur in pregnancies. No, it's not 'normal', but how many of us are?

Year 4, Tuesday 26 February—
More bad news

I am on my back with a foetal heart monitor and a heart full of willing hope. I have nothing but a Doppler machine and the Home and Health Channel on TV. I find it reassuring to watch other people's true stories about pregnancy—it makes me feel not so alone. True to real life TV, I receive a call from a colleague advising me that his wife had just lost her IVF baby at 18 weeks due to an infection in the placenta. We were both in the same stage of pregnancy and would often talk about getting together for play dates and sharing late night bottle sessions. The funeral would be in two weeks, but first his partner has to give birth to the foetus. It is just too devastating for me to hear, whilst lying on my couch, grasping at every little heartbeat and butterfly kick. As I console my friend, I feel guilty for still hanging onto the life inside me. It is desperate times. Things are happening at a faster pace than I am able to process. Now when I need the confidence to get through my own hurdles and deal with the magnitude of what was currently happening to me, I also have to deal with the deepest grief for my friend. After all, I am only a stone's throw away from it myself.

Year 4, Friday 29 February— *Happy Birthday Daddy*

We made it to our 18-week ultrasound. Seeing our babies hearts beating and their little limbs moving around is always such a relief. It also happened to be Fez's 40th birthday, and I knew there would be nothing better to give him for his birthday than finding out the sex of our twins. The bleeding had eased but it is evident on the scan that these little pockets of blood lying above my cervix are something I will just have to live with. They serve as a little reminder of the struggle we went through to make it to this point. It is always there, nudging at my consciousness. It is reassuring to know that the babies are growing normally and are big enough to sustain themselves, should there be any further major blood loss. Medically speaking, we were out of the woods.

By the time we got around to Twin A on the scan, the sonographer had already printed out a tiny take home photo of our 18 week old nugget with the words "Happy Birthday Daddy" printed on the top. She then presented Fez with the photo and told him that his first born will be a son. The tears welled up—once again—and the pride I felt for that image on a flimsy piece of photo paper was incomparable. Twin A is my little boy!

We moved onto the scan for our little nugget number two. Measurements were taken and documented and then the scan stopped abruptly. The sonographer got up and excused herself, saying she would be back in a moment. She needed another doctor's opinion on something. My heart began to pound. What could possibly be wrong now? Here we go, just when the bleeding eases, there is going to be another factor to worry about. I started to break into a sweat.

Within minutes, a doctor who specialises in complicated twin pregnancies came into the room and introduced himself. He had a look at the ultrasound results and explained to us in layman's terms that there was an unfamiliar growth in the abdomen of our little Twin B. The mass was quite a size in comparison to the rest of the 18 week old baby and it is taking up just about all of the stomach area. I immediately thought the worse. A tumour? A growth? Is it sinister? Benign? How will we be able to treat this without sacrificing the welfare of Twin A—our son?

The doctor explained that we would need to have continuous monitoring and that he couldn't offer an accurate explanation as to what the growth could be, other than the possibility of an ovarian cyst that has grown as a result of my blood hormones. This diagnosis is momentarily overshadowed by the realisation that our Twin B is a girl! A pigeon pair. Our nuggets now have their own little identities and we named them there and then—Ayden and Kiana. I felt that giving them a name would give them an existence and despite any sinister outcome arising from this latest hurdle, would mean they were alive and very much already a part of our living world. It would be harder to take them away from me if they had a name. They were real.

On the way home, we both had a nagging anxiety over our little girl's cyst, but we owed it to ourselves to celebrate and purchase our first official baby item. I was tired of these great moments always being tainted with bad news. We avoided all the cute baby clothes and purchased a rocking chair for the nursery. It was a safe purchase.

Year 4, Tuesday 18 March— 20 Weeks

We are technically half-way through the pregnancy and there is still a cloud looming over our heads. I still can't bring myself to buy baby clothes yet. That would be too painful to deal with if we didn't make it. Having dealt with so much disappointment along the way has completely destroyed my trust in anything being final. There is never a worry-free moment but I tell you what, those tiny first happy birthday photos of our nuggets were distributed all over the house. I even sent one to mum and dad to put on their fridge.

I've hired another singer to fill in for me for band gigs. I can't afford to be on my feet for long periods of time, risking more blood loss and premature delivery. I spend most of my time on the internet and talking on the phone to mum. The business brings in enough income to sustain us and my hiatus is not forever. I just have to take it easy and I'm not taking any chances.

Year 4, Thursday 27 March—
9 years

The following week mum and dad arrived in Sydney for a belated birthday celebration for Fez. It was also our ninth wedding anniversary. It had always been my dream for Fez to be a father by the time he was 40. It had brought me such sadness to think he would never experience fatherhood. What an amazing way to toast my wonderful husband, on his 40th year and our nine years of marriage.

As a surprise for my parents, we organised another ultrasound so that mum and dad could accompany us and see their grandchildren move for the first time. The experience was surreal. There were tears running down my mum's face as she witnessed the miracle of life tumbling and turning on the screen in front of her. There are not many moments in life that can top this.

The doctor explained that Kiana's (Twin B's) cyst had continued to grow but was still consistent with being an ovarian cyst. If the cyst didn't dissipate on its own, it was possible she may need surgery when she is born. I guess we just have to deal with that when the time comes. For the moment, I am just focused on getting them here safe and sound and meeting my two little nuggets face to face.

The doctor explained that the worst case scenario in the long term for Kiana's ovarian cyst is that she could be infertile due to extensive damage to her ovaries. The news hit me like a brick to the head. Here I am, experiencing a life with unexplained infertility and now I will possibly have to explain to my daughter that she too may suffer this horrendous path in life. The irony of it all is that I was the one who caused it. It is my maternal hormones that have gone into overdrive to produce two babies which consequently affected her tiny little ovaries. The guilt, even for a tiny foetus, is significant enough to make me physically sick.

Year 4, Wednesday 9 April—
23 Weeks

Two weeks later and I am still sick. This unexplained sickness means another trip to my OB and another scan. The diagnosis is that Kiana's cyst has now grown to 10 cms. Dr Van Der Griend pencils in an elective Caesarian at 37 weeks and, although Ayden is head down, Kiana is breech and it is uncertain if the sheer size of this cyst would impact on her breathing when born. It is confirmed as the best birth plan. 37 weeks is generally considered full term for twins. There are still so many of those dreaded 'what ifs'. But I have made it to over half way. I've had to contend with unexplained bleeding, Kiana's growing cyst, falling ill, excruciating ligament pain as my tummy grows bigger and bigger, and I still feel doubly blessed.

Year 4, Sunday 22 June—
34 Weeks

I've made it. Dr. Van der Griend called to say they have pushed my C section back a week as he will be away on holidays in my scheduled 37th week. So my new date was now pencilled in to be at 38 weeks and one day. I joked with Dr Van der Griend that he was prolonging my pregnancy anxiety but he assured me I could carry my twins for the extra week. There are certainly no signs of them wanting to go anywhere yet. I've been fortunate.

As the final weeks pass, I forgive my infertility demons and even manage to allow myself the pure pleasure of having my very own baby shower. This doesn't come without reservations. The last time I over enthusiastically announced to the world that I was pregnant was when I ended up in the emergency ward at RPA hospital, severely heamorrhaging. I am still somewhat plagued by that experience, even at this late stage in the pregnancy, I feel it could all be pulled from under me at any given time. Nothing is ever for certain.

So as I contemplated the thought of my own baby shower I remembered what got me through in those very early days—the little red polka dotted dress. I had just about forgotten about it, hanging idly there in my expanding maternity wardrobe. I arranged for a few of my closest girlfriends to come over and before I could give it a second thought, I was the guest of honour at my very own baby shower—wearing that very same red polka dot. Behind all the generous gifts and perfectly iced cup cakes, is the biggest gift of all. The gift of hope, to never give up when everything does fail, and the knowledge that you just have to hang onto whatever gets you through at the time.

Year 4, Friday 18 July—
My miracle(s)

On the 18th of July, we welcomed into the world Twin A—Ayden Vernon Krizak and Twin B—Kiana Joan Ruzarka Krizak at 8.16 am and 8.17 am respectively. Ayden's middle name, Vernon, is in honour of my father and Kiana is given mum's middle name Joan, as well as Fez's 85 year old grandmother's name Ruzarka. Ayden is the older brother by just one minute—a fact that I was sure would become a teasing point in years to come.

There is something about the history in their names that cements this journey for us. My babies are wrapped and handed to me in one unbelievable moment. I hold them to my chest and feel their first breaths of life. The battle to get them here remains close to my heart, but they are both beautiful, and healthy, and weigh in at 3.3 kilos each. It is an extraordinary end to a very long 38 weeks and one day.

What seems like an effortless feat for so many others in life is my proudest struggle. I guess what it has taught me the most is that sometimes it is worth giving every inch of yourself to fulfil your dreams. Even in the constant face of adversity, I was one of the lucky ones. Even if I had failed, I am not sure I would have looked at it as a failure in the long term. I needed to know I had given my all and I know I would have been comfortable with that. The emotion would never have left us I'm sure, but we would have eventually accepted our path and got on with making the most out of our lives together.

The thing is, until you experience holding your baby—your own flesh and blood—in your arms, totally dependent on you for life, you really don't have any idea what it was that you didn't have. In that sense, I think ignorance is bliss.

In a world where we celebrate the news of abundant pregnant bellies everywhere, I'd like to celebrate all the women and men who have encountered their own infertility journey. Those who have tried and tried again, only to fail in their quest to start a biological family. The experience never leaves you but it is how you choose to use that experience which is empowering to you. You could take it with you through life and learn to love and appreciate what you do have, or choose to be unfulfilled and burdened by grief. I can only urge those of you out there to embrace what's not only behind you, but that which is also before you as you continue life's journey one moment at a time.

We'll never know why we are chosen for this path. Maybe it is to make us see life in a different way. Maybe it is to give us the gift of appreciating the true value of new life and let it impact us in a way that enables us to go the extra mile by reaching out to someone else. You can leave your own mark behind by making a difference in this world, maybe not genetically but spiritually and emotionally.

I've learned that wherever you find your peace, it's important to know that you have done your best in this universe. That the path ahead will continue to be full of many twists and turns, but it all comes down to how we deal with them. We can never control the path but we can choose to control our reactions to the outcome. I can't honestly say 'enjoy the journey' because although the journey can be hard and utterly debilitating at times, you will come out the other end. Perhaps you'll be a little scathed, but still alive and above all else, still grateful for life itself.

CONCLUSION

Just the beginning

Year 6, 26 May

As I sit here writing my final entry for this journal, I'm well aware that it has taken me five years to complete it. I started writing all those years ago as a kind of therapy. It felt good to get it all out when there were times I could barely think, let alone speak. The fear and grief over that time was intense. As I look back now, I haven't forgotten those fears. I've just learnt to deal with them. Every time I look into my babies eyes, I recall the struggle to get them here like it was just yesterday.

I still feel guilty when the sheer demands of motherhood overwhelm me. I wanted this, I made it happen, but no one could ever have prepared me for how hard it is. It's those times when I have to dig deep and still give thanks by remembering where I've come from and where all of this started.

It's been two years since the twins were born and, of course, they are completely oblivious to how they came into this world. Kiana's cyst eventually dissipated six weeks after birth but with this comforting news came another blow. At her seven week paediatric follow up, she was diagnosed with congenital hip dysplasia and spent most of her infant life in full body plaster, unable to move until her completely dislocated hips had fused back together. I never got to hold her close for the first seven months of her life and, to this day, I still feel sad for not only missing out on bonding, skin to skin, but for Ayden who was often left waiting as his sister's needs were put before his. One day I will explain all of this to them.

In the future, I hope to have the courage to give them this book on their 18th birthday, with my greatest wish being for them to discover, through my words on these pages, just how loved they are. When I think about what the next 16 years of life has in store for them, I have such mixed emotions. I'm scared. Scared of the unknown, of what the future holds and how on earth there will ever come a day when I will kiss my children goodbye and send them off into this big, uncertain world.

I loved you before you were mine. I loved you before your heart started beating. I waited so long to meet you and, at times I just didn't know when or how. But now it's so clear. If I had not waited, I wouldn't have you. And it is you that is the perfect soul for me. It was you that I was waiting for and it was worth every living moment. I love you my dear child.

Happy Birthday,
Your Mum

ACKNOWLEDGEMENTS

There are so many people I'd like to acknowledge that have helped make this book possible. Namely the people who have taken my dream from paper to a reality—The staff, doctors and scientists at GENEA Sydney. Lindsay Gillan for being the first person to pick up my manuscript and believe that my story could help others. I am eternally grateful to you. Kate Carruthers for your support and also for believing in my story. Michael Campbell for being brave enough to work with me on the first of 9 edits and helping to get me to one of many next levels! Jen Pope for your wonderful editing and always putting me and my story first. Dr Mark Livingstone for helping me achieve my ultimate dream. My girlfriends who were there to not only listen and hear me whine, but to pick me up and offer support when I needed it most. My dear Mum who shadowed me in the process and shared every imaginable emotion along the way. To the anonymous bloggers around the world whose words and shared stories in the dark of the lonely night meant more to me than I could ever express. Lisa Hanrahan for your guided help and support. And lastly, to the man who was there to witness every word lived on these pages—My husband Fez. You never gave up and you didn't falter when I suggested we try again and again. I never thought I'd ever say this but we are the luckiest people in the world. Thank you.

Q & A ON TRYING TO CONCEIVE

Courtesy of Genea World Leaders in Fertility

What is infertility?

Infertility is the inability of a couple to achieve conception after about a year of unprotected intercourse, or the inability to carry pregnancies to a live birth. Many couples suffering infertility problems can be successfully treated with medical or surgical techniques, or lifestyle changes.

What's the best age to have a baby?

What's best is what's right for you but, the fact is, as you get older it does become harder to conceive. By 35, the chance of a woman conceiving each month is decreased by almost half from the time that she was her most fertile, in her early 20s. There are a number of reasons why some women delay starting a family. The important thing is to be aware, informed and realistic about the age-related decline in fertility.

We're still trying to conceive while many of my friends conceive first time. Why?

First rule of parenting: never compare yourself to anyone else! Everyone's unique so it can happen immediately or take a while longer. Remember that the list of what constitutes 'normal' is a long as a piece of string.

So when should I start worrying?

If you're having regular, unprotected sex and actively trying to get pregnant for more than a year without success then it's a good idea to make an appointment to see your doctor. However, if you're over 35, think about taking a trip to your GP after six months of trying.

I've already had a baby, does that mean I will conceive easily second time around?

Unfortunately, not always. About 10 per cent of couples with children will experience trouble conceiving again—known as **secondary infertility**.

What are some of the medical causes of infertility?

- blocked or damaged fallopian tubes
- low sperm count or problems with sperm function
- severe endometriosis
- ovarian problems that prevent the production or release of eggs
- uterine abnormalities, such as an irregular shaped uterus or fibroids

So, the problem isn't always with the woman?

No, in about 40 per cent of cases where couples have trouble conceiving, the problem lies with the man. It's normally the quality or quantity of sperm that affects his fertility. Equally, about 40 per cent of infertility is linked to female issues such as absence or irregularity of ovulation or blocked fallopian tubes. In the remaining 20 per cent, the cause of infertility problems are not identified—known as **unexplained infertility**.

Does unexplained infertility mean we'll never have a baby?

Not necessarily. One in six Australian couples suffer infertility but, of these, about one in five have what's known as idiopathic (unexplained) infertility, where there is no explanation of why a couple can't conceive.

What is IVF?

When IVF was first developed, people talked about 'test tube' babies. But 'in vitro' means 'in glass' and the process involves bringing eggs and sperm together in a glass or plastic dish in a lab. Any procedure where fertilisation takes place outside the body is a form of IVF.

How does it work?

Every month, follicles begin to develop in a woman's ovaries. Around one to 30 follicles will grow each menstrual cycle—depending on a woman's age. But just one follicle will dominate and release a mature egg.

During an IVF cycle, injections of a hormone known as FSH (Follicle Stimulating Hormone) are used to encourage more of the follicles to develop mature eggs—which are then collected under vaginal ultrasound guidance—sometimes called OPU, egg pick up or retrieval.

The eggs are then fertilised in the lab. The developing embryos are monitored for several days, before one is transferred to the uterus. If there are additional embryos, they can be frozen and stored for later use.

What are the chances of IVF success?

Many factors contribute to any couple's chance of success, including age. But Genea has a long history of providing the best possible chance of having a healthy baby. And the birth rate among Genea's patients is more than 30 per cent higher, per embryo transfer, than the average of other clinics in Australia and New Zealand, according to data from the Australian Institute of Health and Welfare.[*]

On average how many cycles does it take to get pregnant?

This will vary between clinics, and success rates will also be affected by the age of the woman undertaking IVF. At Genea, almost 60 per cent of our patients overall will have a baby. And 90 per cent of these women will have a baby within three or less cycles of IVF. Unfortunately, this chance drops significantly in women over 40.

I hate needles, do I have to inject myself?

Most IVF drugs do not work when taken orally, so injections will be required. Modern IVF drugs are for the most part packaged in pen-like devices, similar to insulin pens that diabetics use. If you are very uncomfortable with injecting

---

[*]   Figures based on 2010 AIHW data, published October 2012

yourself other options can be sought such as your partner or a friend administering the injections.

Do the drugs have side effects?

Many women will feel a little bloated and tender in the lower abdomen before and after the egg collection. Other common side effects may include breast tenderness, nausea, and headaches. Mood changes can occur but they are not universal. Genea offers a counselling service to all couples going through IVF.

How long does a cycle take?

This will depend on the type of treatment you are having and your individual response to the medication. On average it takes between 8-14 days of FSH injections before the egg collection procedure takes place. There's then 2-5 days until the embryo is transferred into the uterus, and 10-14 days before your period is expected.

Will stress affect my chance of pregnancy?

Luckily there is no indication that stress negatively affects the chance of pregnancy with IVF. (Not only is this the case 'anecdotally', but a recent, formal research study from Sweden also showed no harmful correlation between level of stress and IVF success rates.) But the more stressed you are the more difficult the experience of IVF is likely to be. At Genea, our nurses and counsellors are there to help you during this time.

Does IVF increase my chance of having twins?

Historically, the link between IVF treatment and multiple pregnancies was due to more than one embryo being transferred back to the uterus. However, as IVF technologies have improved, there has been a move towards single embryo transfer. If only one embryo is transferred the chance of twins is about 1 per cent because of an embryo splitting to cause an identical twin pregnancy. This is much lower than other forms of assisted reproduction. Genea first introduced routine single embryo transfer in 1996 and now approximately 80 per cent of all embryo transfers undertaken at Genea's clinics involve the return of a single embryo, regardless of patient age, and only five per cent of patients have a multiple birth. The multiple birth rate for IVF patients across Australia and New Zealand is 8.2 per cent, [according to the 2009 ANZARD data published in November 2011.]

How soon will I know if I'm pregnant?

Pregnancy can be confirmed using blood tests about 13 days after egg aspiration. An ongoing pregnancy can be confirmed by ultrasound 3 weeks after this.

Do I need a break between cycles?

It's usually wise to have at least one month's break following a stimulated IVF cycle, but you can go "back-to-back" if you're doing a natural or frozen embryo transfer IVF cycle.

Is the transfer of a frozen embryo less likely to result in a pregnancy?

At Genea, success rates from frozen embryos are now on a par with fresh embryos. Currently, patients have a frozen embryo transfer either following a fresh transfer that did not develop into a pregnancy, or when they are trying for another baby following a successful fresh transfer and they have frozen embryos in storage.

Genea was the first Australian clinic group to introduce 'snap freezing' vitrification as a standard practice in 2006. And more than 1,000 babies have been born to Genea patients after the transfer of frozen embryos. More than 95 per cent of embryos that are snap frozen survive the vitrification and warming processes.

Almost 50 per cent of frozen embryo transfers in Genea patients aged less than 38 will result in a pregnancy. That compares to a success rate of less than 25 per cent just five years ago.

Can lifestyle factors, such as exercise and nutrition affect fertility?

Being overweight or obese has been proven not only to reduce the chances of a couple conceiving naturally, but also means fertility treatment, such as IVF, is less likely to be successful.

The good news is that fertility is improved with a relatively modest degree of weight loss or gain. But with hectic lifestyles and so many weight loss messages out there, it might be difficult to know what is right for you.

Genea's Top ten fertility tips

1. Don't leave it too late! Women are born with all their eggs and they decline in both quantity and quality over time. As a result, the chance of a woman conceiving drops sharply in the late 30s to early 40s.

2. Formulate a good diet and exercise routine. Women have a higher chance of conception when they are in a normal body mass index range and either if either partner is overweight or obese, the chances of pregnancy are reduced considerably. In both men and women a BMI of 18.5-24.9 is considered normal weight.

3. Take appropriate preconception supplements. All women trying to conceive should take supplemental folic acid (folate) to ensure the best chance of a healthy pregnancy. Many women are also deficient in vitamin D and iodine.

4. Know your cycle. Women with 28 day menstrual cycles usually ovulate midway between their menses—about 14 days after the start of their period. There are various simple methods of determining when you ovulate. This time— and slightly earlier—is the best time to have unprotected sex.

5. Don't (or stop) smoking and significantly curtail alcohol and caffeine consumption. Smoking is toxic to human eggs and has long lasting negative effects even after a woman stops.

6. Make sure your other half is also well and healthy, is not smoking and also reducing alcohol intake. It takes two to tango.

7. Try to have sex about every other day, particularly leading up to the middle of your cycle.

8. Remember that your friends—and even your mother—are not necessarily fertility experts despite their personal experiences. Their advice might be well meaning, but not necessarily accurate.

9. Try to relax. Obsessing about conception can be counterproductive and leave you stressed. Consider any strategies that reduce anxiety and help you remain positive.

10. Live a normal and happy life. There is no evidence that you need to reduce normal levels of exercise or somehow wrap yourself in cotton wool while you are trying to conceive.

'Q & A ON TRYING TO CONCEIVE'
courtesy of Genea World Leaders in Fertility

www.genea.com.au

If you need more advice Genea has a Fertility Advisor who is available for a complimentary consultation to discuss the variety of treatment options available to you, costs and success rates. This is not a medical appointment, but an opportunity for you to ask questions, gain more information and help you select the right service or fertility specialist.

In Australia, call 1300 361 795 to book an appointment or go to our website.